Norma,
I loved meeting you!!
You are beautiful inside + out.
Live a superfantastic life everyday.
Love

Laura London
XOXO

HOT AND HEALTHY BODY

BY LAURA LONDON

LIFECHANGE PRESS

AMSTERDAM

Special Thanks To My Amazing Photographers

Mike Brochu – Cover Photo

Chuck Hersh Photography – Inside Photos

Claude Taylor, Goodlivin Productions – Author Photo

Dedication

This book is dedicated to:

Women and mothers all over the world who give of themselves, tirelessly and with love from the heart. I thank you for letting me be a part of your fitness and wellness journey. I acknowledge you for having the deep desire and passion to improve the quality of your life and of the ones you love.

Big thank you to my husband and my 3 wonderful children for letting me be me. My Mom for making me have great posture and letting me be a free spirit and supporting me always.

I could not do what I do without the support and constant encouragement of my husband Adam, "Mr. London". He is constantly there with a big smile and always full of excitement with each new opportunity that comes our way. He picks me up when I am down, knows what I am thinking without me even saying a word. He is my husband, my rock and my best friend.

My children have watched me go from "Mom" to "Super Mom with Muscles". It has been an adjustment to say the least. Thank you for your patience and understanding when I am on the computer 24/7. For giving me your support and your love. There is nothing I cherish more in the world than the three of you.

Lastly, to my three best friends in the whole world, Sally, Dawn and Jan, without whom I could not do life. They have supported, encouraged and loved me through all the ups and downs that life brings. Having you three in my life has made me a better wife, mom and friend. I love you all dearly.

Laura

Table of Contents

Foreword

I am so glad you are here! I have created the "Hot & Healthy Body" program just for you, whether you are a mom, aunt, daughter, fitness diva or newbie or just plain sick and tired of being sick and tired. I am here for you.

I have been blessed to have the opportunity to meet and speak with people all over the world about health, nutrition and exercise and learn from each of them.

Why do I work out, Why do I push myself day after day when there are so many other things I could be doing with my time?

Why do I make the time between 3 kids, a husband, pets, running my own business, homework and carpools?

Because I was tired of being tired, feeling depressed and wondering if this is all life was supposed to be. I wanted to be in control of my life and my body again. Getting into shape has been an amazing life altering journey for me full of personal growth, as well as giving me a deep knowledge of myself and what I am capable of if I put my mind to it.

We all have the power to change our lives, to live healthier, happier and love more. If you want it, you can have it.

You just have to want it bad enough and you will find a way to get it.

Friends, I know that together we can improve the quality of your life, get in shape and have fun at the same time.

I wrote this book to help you break weight loss down and make it simple. There is so much information out there, I think we get information overload.

Losing weight should not have to be so complicated. We all know that cutting calories way too low and starving ourselves does not work, nor does doing endless amounts of cardio. There has to be a better way and it starts with nutrition and what you put into your body.

I have spent a lot of time and hard work studying, researching and experimenting on my own body. I read each new fitness and nutrition book that comes out on the market. I have lived as a figure competitor, vegetarian, vegan and even a raw foodist. I love to learn about each new diet and how it affects the body.

I am a mom of three with a busy schedule just like you and don't have time to spend hours in the gym or plan and count every calorie that goes into my body.

This nutrition program is the way I live my life every day and it works. Read through all the information and then let it soak in. Listen to your inner voice because you really do know what to do.

I am just here to help guide you along the way.

Aren't you frustrated getting fitness advice from a young girl who is half your age and who has zero experience in LIFE?

Most fitness gurus have never had to deal with any of the fitness, metabolism and time management issues of a woman who is experienced and has balanced a life full of kids, family, and career.

If you want to increase your energy, ignite your confidence, lose weight and be in charge of your health, then keep reading.

My nutrition plan will teach you how to eat healthy for life. To stop the endless diets and disappointments that come with them.

I teach you a solid foundation that you can use in your everyday life to make eating easier and do-able.

We are all busy, actually, non-stop and always on the go. We need to make our daily nutrition quick and easy so we can get to all the other things we busy moms and women need to do.

These principles can be applied not only to you but to your family as well. I am not going to tell you what to eat every day. I want you to understand how to create your meals so they are flavorful, exciting and packed with nutrition.

If I give you meal plans to follow, you will never truly understand how to create your own meals and be super successful. I give you the guidelines and ""Nutritional Laws" to follow so you can plan and prepare for success.

This is my Hot and Healthy Eating bible. The plan that helps me keep my nutrition and body in check year round.

I believe in the 90% / 10% rule. See how I use it to never feel deprived, keep my cravings in check and live a healthy lifestyle.

You already know that you're fabulous, but you need someone who can show you how to discover and become an even better version of yourself - because they have done it themselves. Who doesn't want to feel more CONFIDENT, SEXY, and POWERFUL? Let's get started now.

- Laura London

My Story

If you ever told me I would be writing a book, I would have said no way not ever. Least of all a health and wellness book. Well... guess what? I am! So here we go....

I truly believe that everyone is here on this earth for a certain purpose. Sometimes we know it right away and sometimes it takes us a lifetime to figure out. Well, I fall right there in the middle I found my purpose and my passion at 43.

Let's rewind and start at the beginning of this story. I came into this world and was adopted when I was only five days old. The way I have always looked at being adopted is that I was a "special" child and was put into this family for a reason. That reason, I believe has become part of my journey.

I was adopted by a wonderful family, who were European immigrants. My father was French and my mother was English.

My brother was two years older than I. He had been diagnosed with Hemophilia, a rare blood condition where your blood does not clot. My parents were told if they had another child there would be a 50% chance that child would have Hemophilia too.

So, in came little Laura to this family.

Growing up, my brother was always on crutches, in and out of hospitals and almost daily had to inject himself with needles and clotting factor to survive. Needless to say my house was a very serious place. I think that is when I decided at a young age I wanted to blend in and be safe, not cause any problems and try to make everyone around me happy. This may sound strange, but I almost felt guilty for being the "healthy" child. I saw my brother suffer so much and my parents do everything in their power to help him. They donated blood every week at the blood bank.

Let's fast forward. My brother went to college and I was in high school. The only thing was I kept falling asleep in school and no one knew why. Then, finally after numerous doctor visits, medications and tests, I was diagnosed with Mononucleosis. It was so bad my parents had to take me out of school and brought me to Florida and the warm sunshine to recuperate. I had never been this sick in my life. I was barely able to move my body and my skin was ghostly white. I remember not even being able to lift my arms up. It was very scary. My throat was practically closed up and it was hard to even breath. My glands were extremely swollen. It took me over a month to recuperate, but I did get better and kept living life.

I went on to college, where I was living the life. Studying, drinking, and smoking cigarettes. I was sleep deprived and my eating habits were out of control; talk about the freshman 15 and then some! They used to call me "candy girl" because I always had some kind of candy in my pockets.

Well don't you know, I kept getting sick. I went from doctor to doctor. They would prescribe all sorts of medication but I never felt better. Finally, I went to see a very special Dr. in New York City and was diagnosed with Chronic Fatigue and Epstein Barr and a systemic yeast overgrowth in my bloodstream.

This doctor did something no one else had ever done. He told me to change my eating habits! Put me on a special diet, high quality nutritional supplements and special allergy type shots, and monitored my results. I had to travel over an hour every month to go and see him. Slowly I got better, my extreme fatigue, fuzzy thinking and overall health got better. This was great! And life went on, until…

My brother, who was in college now, and may I brag at MIT as a computer engineer was diagnosed with HIV due to a bad blood transfusion. The blood companies that supplied the clotting factor that he needed to live, did not do an extra step to clean the tainted blood clotting factor and in turn infected 10,000 Hemophiliacs, who in turn infected their wives and their children. Had my brother not suffered enough his whole life with this disease, and now HIV unnecessarily? He went from a healthy vibrant young man, into a sick, frail, and pharmaceutical drug dependent victim. Michael was a strong person and never complained and kept going.

I got married and then was expecting my first child when things came crashing down around me. When I was nine months pregnant my father died unexpectedly. My father was the rock of our family. He took care of me and my brother, as well as his mother and his brother who had a stroke in his early forties. I had to run his real estate office. I went from being the secretary to being the president of his company overnight. I received power of attorney for his mom, my grandmother, and had to make all her medical decisions, put her in a nursing home all the while having my first baby. I remember pushing my grandmother down the hallway in her wheelchair with one arm and pushing the stroller with my other. I was always crying, from having a newborn and the lack of sleep, the death of my father, running his company, and the responsibility of my grandmother and my sick brother were tremendous. I also put on well over 40 pounds due to depression.

On top of all this I finally found my birth mother who I had been searching for since I was a teenager. But that, my friends, is another book in itself. But needless to say it was quite an emotional time for me. I always say you do not know how strong you really are until you need to be.

You never know what or whom life will send to you when you need them most. I was sent an angel that helped me through this extremely hard time. She may not even realize it but I don't think I could have gotten through this time without her.

Her name is Lucy and I met her in my Lamaze class at the hospital. Lucy was deaf and had a hearing baby. We became good friends and I loved learning to sign with her so much that I enrolled in a program to study to be an interpreter for the deaf. Lucy would take care of my baby whenever I had to go to class or go to a board meeting for my father's business. Sign language gave me an outlet, something to focus on instead of losing my dad.

But I had a small baby and had to keep moving forward. I never had a chance to breathe let alone grieve for my father. Then I was diagnosed with some pre-cancerous cells that sent me on a healing journey.

I went and studied with Brenda Cobb from the Living Foods in Atlanta and learned all about raw foods, sprouting, wheatgrass, colon cleansing and emotional healing. I read every book I could get my hands on about nutrition. I was looking and feeling the best I had ever felt in my life. I lived the raw lifestyle until I moved to Florida from Connecticut.

I kept going, never ever slowing down. I had two more babies in a very short amount of time. The doctor told me I was having a girl and it turned out to be a boy! That was quite a shocker. One of my children was also on the autistic spectrum and did not like to be held or touched very much. I enrolled in a reflexology course thinking this would be a great way to have some connection, but it turns out the child was ticklish! But I still loved the reflexology class and it gave me an outlet and something to focus on.

One day, out of the blue, I got the phone call that my brother had passed away during the night. He went to the hospital alone in the middle of the night and then he was gone. How much more could I take; my father, and now my only sibling, my brother. Life was very cruel to him. I will never forget being on vacation with him and knowing that he was eventually going to die. He asked me if I would take care of mom and dad for him. It was heart-breaking to say the least.

Now I became the president of my brother's Internet Company with three small kids. I know nothing about the Internet. I miss the simple days when I woke up, went to work, and came home. Life just kept going and I kept going. Never grieving, never taking the time to take care of myself mentally, physically or emotionally.

One day I was grocery shopping. I will never forget it.

I had a long housecoat type dress on with baby spit-up on each shoulder; I was at least 40 lbs. overweight and tired. I picked up a fitness magazine with before and after transformations in it. Now you have to realize I had never EVER seen anything like this before. I never played a sport growing up because of my brother's Hemophilia; we never even watched sports on TV. I was what you call "sports illiterate".

I was amazed at what I was seeing, page after page of physique transformations. I decided, still not quite sure why or what possessed me but I decided I was going to do that too! Now, I am a Taurus and we Tauruses are very stubborn so when we get an idea in our brain there is no stopping us.

I joined the gym with my shirt covering my body down to my knees. I wrote down my goals in a journal. I wrote down what I was going to eat, the exercises I was going to do at the gym. I posted motivational pictures around the house. I read more about health and nutrition. I turned my car into a mobile university. I was determined to transform. But this way of "bodybuilding eating" was very different from my green organic lifestyle. But I thought OK, I am going to do everything they say to do for 90 days and see what happens. Realize I did not miss a workout or a meal. I gave it 110%. Do you know what happened? The fat came off, muscles started to appear. I replaced my long T-shirt at the gym with cropped tops and people were asking me what the heck I was doing.

I met a trainer at the gym who took me under her wing. She was a fitness competitor and I had recognized her from Oxygen magazine. The sport of Figure was brand new and she introduced me to the sport of figure competing. Now, I have three left feet, meaning coordination is not my thing. I never even danced until I went to college. I could barely manage the 4 quarter turns that I had to do on stage. I still don't know what gives me the courage to step so far out of my comfort zone, but I did it and I got on stage and won first place three times. It was a lot of work and a lot of fun and a major accomplishment in my life.

I wish the story ended here but I have to share this with you. After each competition, my body broke down. I would get strep throat and wanted to eat everything in sight because I had denied myself "nutritious food" over "competition food". Then life got in the way. I stopped competing and now had no outside personal goal and life came crashing down on me. I had been going full steam ahead since my father and brother had died, finding my birth mother, and caring for my grandmother. I never ever took the time to grieve, to cry or to deal with my internal emotions.

My life was way out of control, I became very depressed, and food was my comfort. I would make excuses to go to the grocery store for milk when I knew I was really going for a candy bar or two. To top it off I had a back injury now that was causing me severe pain and I was even having trouble walking because of it. My whole body and system was sick, emotionally and physically. My body was screaming at me but I was not listening.

I packed on 40 lbs. pounds again and a few years went by. I knew I needed help when I found myself throwing up into a cup in my car all alone and crying. I called my three best friends in the world and told them I needed help. I could not have gotten through this without them and my loving husband and mother. It was time to deal with the deaths of the two most important men in my life and the fact that I had finally found the birth mother I had been searching for for years.

Fast forward to 43. I woke up with my hormones out of control, addicted to sugar, fat where I never had it before and doing a weight loss program online. Did I mention the pants with the elastic waistband? How the heck did I get here? I was embarrassed because I had been in such good shape a few years before and now it was overwhelming to try to lose that weight for the second time.

I made the decision in my head. I said, oh heck NO! This is not what the 40's and the rest of my life are going to be like, and that one decision has changed the course of my life in my 40's.

I started walking at first because that is all my back would let me do, and then I joined the gym. I started to eat healthy, green and organic again, going back to what I truly believed in a more plant based diet. I worked hard, carefully and slowly and got in shape again, which is not as easy to do in your 40's. I got up the courage to get back on stage. This time the "healthy green way" and I have not looked back since.

Remember at the beginning of this story when I said we are all here for a special purpose? I now know my purpose. It is to inspire and motivate you to be your best at any age and step out of your comfort zone to live your true life's purpose. Life begins outside of your comfort zone. Trust me on this!

Hot & Healthy Mindset 101

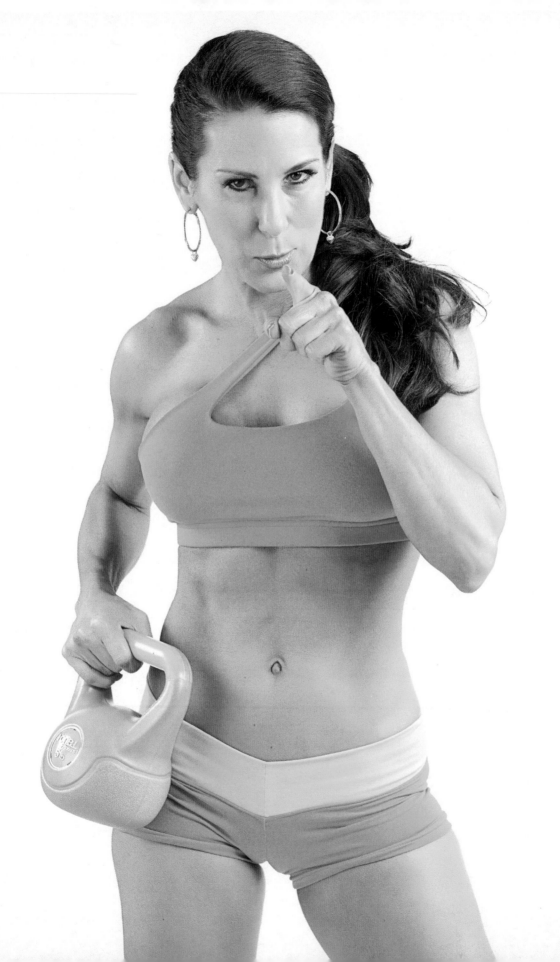

Awakening The Power Within

Fitness is the first key component to awakening the POWER within you for transformation, and usually it is the most difficult to fit into a busy lifestyle.

I believe that you don't need to schedule hours of extra time every day to achieve good fitness goals. Exercise can become part of your daily life in ways that don't require crazy time commitments.

I am known as the Green Fitness Goddess for a good reason, and I share all the nutrition tips you will ever need to eat healthy food that not only tastes great, but also won't leave you feeling bad about yourself later. I believe that the right foods will fuel the body and the mind. Taking control of your health and wellness means taking control of your kitchen - and stepping away from the takeout!

The Hot and Healthy Body Program can be done at home or in the gym. You can do anything for 30 days! Just make the decision and do it, and do it for yourself.

Muscle burns 300 times more calories at rest than fat! WOW, that is pretty AMAZING... That is why doing endless amounts of cardio backfire. It is the muscle you want to focus on for fat burning, toning, shaping and tightening. The workouts are based on compound movements so you get your cardio and weight training in at the same time. Talk about a bang for your exercise buck!

The program can be done at home or in the gym. You will need a mat, a set of dumbbells and a stability ball to do these workouts at home.

"Train Like a Woman, Feel Like a Woman, Because You Are a Woman"

~Laura London ~

Ten Steps to Prepare for Success

Take your time and read through these 10 steps because they, along with your WHY are the foundation of the program. If we don't start with a plan and a goal how will we know where we want to go? You don't decide to hop in a car and go on vacation without a plan and you should not do the same thing when it comes to your health and fitness.

Go grab a cup of green tea curl up on the couch and read through the 10 Steps to Prepare for Success. Let them sink in and realize that doing this is just as important if not more than what you eat and how you exercise. These steps are an important part of the Hot and Healthy Body.

1. Change your mindset – This is not a diet, but a way of life that will teach you the tools you need to be successful not only in your health and fitness journey but in all areas of your life.

Ok, ladies it is time to throw away that negative inner talk. You know what I am talking about, "My arms are fat", "I will never be fit", "I am big boned" I don't have the time to exercise", "I am too old". What have you been telling yourself that your brain is believing?

If you are telling your mind this day after day, do you know what is going to happen? Your mind is going to believe it. Your brain can be trained just like your muscles. If you are "training your brain with negative self talk, thoughts of hopelessness or unsuccessfulness then guess what? That is what your brain is going to give you.

I want you to stop and write down some of your OLD negative self-talk. Look at them; read them, do you seriously believe them? Where did they come from? You know they are not true, right? They are only thoughts.

OLD NEGATIVE SELF TALK:

1. _____

2. _____

3. _____

"Don't Believe Everything You Think"

Ok, now that you wrote them down, I want you to cross them out, scribble on them and get mad at them, yell at them if you want. NOW it is time to kick those OLD thoughts to the curb, lets step on them, crush them and say adios bucko! It's time to let them go.

Let's train the brain, work it out just like you would your muscles. At first it may be uncomfortable, maybe even feel a little bit funny but after training your brain to think positive, uplifting thoughts, things start to happen. Just like muscles that start to get stronger, so will your NEW beliefs in what you can do and will accomplish.

Here is an exercise you can do for your brain, that when practiced will wind up burning more calories than you could ever have imagined. Now just like exercise you have to be consistent and persistent. Doing it once is not going to work.

Make this your work, your #1 priority. It is worth it and it's calorie free!

It's Mind Muscle WORKOUT TIME

I call these SLAMMERS. Every time you have one of those OLD negative thoughts, they are sneaky and will try to come back. You are going to SLAM it with a positive thought and mental mind image. BAM!!!! SLAM. Kick it back to the curb.

Find a new mantra or "LIFTER". This is a saying that you will use that motivates you and makes you feel empowered. Here are some suggestions. But really, really do this. Scream one of these "LIFTERS" out loud when you are alone and see how you feel. I want to be able to hear you from my house!

I can do anything!

I am AWESOME!

I LOVE my fit and health body!

I am in charge of my life!

I am Powerful!

> *"Whether you believe you can, or believe you can't,*
> *you are correct!"*
>
> *~ Henry Ford ~*

2. Be true to your word – To succeed, you must follow through with your word. You are making a commitment to yourself and you must keep it for life. If you stray off your path, immediately acknowledge it and move forward. It is O.K, and then move on.

Don't be the one who thinks, I blew it, I will start again on Monday. Do you know what happens to these women? Monday comes and goes and then another Monday comes and goes and then they find that 6 months or a year has gone by.

What I am here to teach you is a lifestyle not a diet, not a quick fix to lose 10 or 20 lbs. and then gain back again. HECK NO!!! I want to give you the power to be in control for the rest of your life. How cool is that!

Take a moment. Are you ready to commit and be true to your word? If you make a promise to someone, I would hope that you are true to your word and keep your promise. So my question is WHY, WHY, WHY would you not keep the promise to yourself?

You are the most important person in your life and deserve to be treated with integrity and respect. You are worth it. So again, if you fall off the wagon, take a wrong turn or even fall flat on your face, it is OK. Don't worry. Just keep moving forward in the direction you are meant to go, FORWARD.

3. PMA – Positive Mental Attitude – This is a journey. It will have ups and downs. BELIEVE that everything is for a reason. You have to experience the downs because they are what give you the motivation to push up and move forward. You can overcome anything. Remain positive even when you feel there is little improvement. Slow and steady wins the race, I promise.

We all know that we do not live in a fairy tale world. Things happen, life, laundry, kids, husbands, jobs, groceries, bills and so much more. It can get quite overwhelming at times. How can we live a healthy life when sometimes it feels like we don't even have a minute to breathe? It's how we learn to deal with what life throws at us that determines our success.

You always have a choice. Always strive to go for the better choice. Choose one small piece of cake instead of 3 pieces, choose 10 minutes of exercise instead of none. Choose calling a friend when you are down instead of crawling in bed and crying.

Take the time to talk to yourself, out-loud or quietly in your head and ask yourself, am I a making the best choice I can make now? Is this choice for my higher good, and will it move me in the direction I want to go?

Sometimes the answer will be yes and sometimes the answer will be no. But just realize you are the one making the choice, no one else.

4. Setting Goals – Set small goals that are attainable. You will reach them and then move on to the next one. Think of them as a ladder taking you rung by rung to get to the top. Keep climbing to the top carefully and you will reach your goals.

The most important step you must take in order to succeed in every area of your life is to identify your goals and put them in writing. Goals left to memory, are goals that easily slip out of mind in the busy-ness of everyday life and responsibilities.

Writing them down makes them real, and a constant reminder of the life-changing journey you have decided to travel on. Reading your goals daily will keep you focused on the steps you must take to make them become a reality. Be as specific as you can on your goal setting. Make sure those goals are realistic and put pressure on yourself by writing deadlines for each one. As you reach your daily and weekly goals you will be building the foundation that will enable you to reach long-term goals. Remember to read your goals everyday for continued inspiration and focus.

Statistics show that people who write down their goals are 80% more successful in achieving them

5. Journaling - Make a commitment to write down your WHY and your goals and read them every day. Log your daily meals, exercise, and how you feel. This is a VERY important step to follow to be successful. It may feel strange at first but the more you write down and journal the more successful you will be. Journaling holds you accountable for what you are or are not doing. I wish I could, but I can't be there with you to make sure you are doing what you need to do every day. Journaling will be your partner and best friend on this health and wellness journey.

6. Make this a priority in your life – Commit to yourself the time, effort and dedication you deserve. Make yourself a priority. When you take the time to take care of you, you will be amazed at what happens around you. Life just seems a little easier.

Why is it we moms/women can make everyone else a priority and if there is any time left over we may do a little something for ourselves? Most of the time we do very little or nothing for ourselves.

Let me share this secret with you. Come in close so you will hear this; YOU ARE A PRIORITY. Did you hear it? If you don't take care of yourself no one else will and you will find yourself in an unhappy place one day and wonder how you got there.

It is so much easier to take off 5 lbs. than 30 lbs. So take the time to take care of you. Doing this will make you feel good, and a happy mom/woman is one of the most beautiful things in the world.

7. Surround yourself with positive people – Let them know how much their support means to you and talk with them when you need a motivation boost. They want to see you succeed. Talk to people who have done what you want to do and ask for their advice. Listen to motivational CD's in the car. Upload them to your phone or IPod and make your car a mobile "KNOWLEDGE UNIVERSITY". I do it all the time and hardly ever listen to music any more. There is too much to learn and discover!

8. Do not give in to excuses – Life will always give you reasons and excuses to not follow through. Don't give in to them, do what you need to do to everyday to reach your goals and honor yourself. You are worth it.

There is always going to be an excuse or reason why you can't do something. I am going to ask you this: Why are some people successful and others are not? We all have excuses or reasons why we CAN'T, but it is the people who do not let them get in the way that are successful. Keep your eye on the prize, focus and push forward to work for what you want.

9. Don't quit and then start over – This is so important! Finish what you start. So many people never achieve the results they want because they never let themselves get far enough. They quit before the results were just about to happen.

It wasn't quick enough for them. It's not about the "quickness". It is about the consistency, planning, follow-through and patience.

One of my favorite quotes a friend shared with me is "Rome was not built in a day, but it is still standing". You want to reach your goal and keep it for life.

"Look inward, you are the expert of you. The moment you stop looking "Out there" for the answers you will become a powerful and confident YOU, who will be in full control of your life."

10. Enjoy the journey – Each of us has our own road to follow, lessons to learn and ups and downs to go through. Slow down, relax and enjoy the journey. The journey is where you will learn much more than losing weight, you will learn about yourself, your desires, beliefs and re-discover who you are along the way. I believe we all have a special unique gift to share with the world. I hope this journey will help you find it and cultivate it to its fullest potential.

Be present in the now, and you will get to where you are meant to be.

~ CHANGE YOUR MIND, CHANGE YOUR BODY,
CHANGE YOUR LIFE ~

~Laura London~

What is your WHY?
Be Clear About it

Before we start the Hot and Healthy Body program we have a big question that needs to be answered. This questions is so important that the whole program is really based around your WHY. In the Hot and Healthy Nutrition and Fitness Journal start to think about and write down your why. Doing this step is key to being successful on the Hot and Healthy Body program.

Why are you doing this program? Is it to lose weight, look better in your clothes, feel more confident? Or maybe it is to improve your health? When we take the time to really find out our WHY we find out other things in the process.

Say your why is to lose 10 pounds for a high school reunion. When you dig deeper into your why, you realize that you want to sleep better or reduce inflammation in your body and that you really want to improve your family's eating habits. Your WHY becomes much bigger and important. When you dig deep and uncover your WHY you may find you have a lot of why's. This is OK. Finding your why will also help you become clearer on setting your goals and how to reach them.

Why do I want to lose 10 pounds?

- To look better in my clothes, to wear cute clothes

- To feel good when I wake up in the morning, to get rid of aches and pains

- To improve my complexion, have shiny hair, long nails

- To help my family eat better, and help them live a healthy life

The great part about writing down and getting really clear on your WHY is that it will evolve. You see from the example above the WHY started out with wanting to lose weight, but what happened along the way were other benefits of losing weight that you may not have thought about.

Visualization

Now that we dug a little deeper about your WHY, we have one more exercise to do before we move on. Napoleon Hill, Author of the book *Think and Grow Rich* said "The first step to reaching your goals is to have a burning desire". It's not enough to just say you want to lose weight and get in shape. You need to have a reason, a burning desire that comes from within yourself. Then you need to develop the skills and an action plan that are going to move you in the directions of your goals. The Hot and Healthy Body has laid out the action steps you need to take. You have to bring the burning desire or, as I like to call it, the fire from within.

Ask yourself what is your burning desire? Am I willing to take the actions steps necessary to get there? Without this important step, a burning desire you are just hoping to get into shape.

Lets talk about what your burning desire feels like. What is it that our souls are truly seeking? Are we truly seeking weight loss or are we seeking the feeling that weight loss will bring about to our soul? What will it feel like when you reach your goal weight?

Will you feel happy, confident, strong, sexy, unstoppable, fierce, bold, radiant, successful or motivated? What we are truly seeking is a feeling because we are emotional beings.

Visualization is the key that will increase your belief in achieving your goals significantly and it helps you believe that you deserve your goals and that they are attainable. Plus it just feels great!

Take 10 - 20 minutes a day and visualize yourself achieving your goals, really feel what it feels like to accomplish them. Write down in your journal what is coming up for you. When we feel it we will become it.

Stop here and write down your WHY in the Hot and Healthy Nutrition and Fitness Journal. Find some alone time and practice visualizing and truly feeling your goals. Take your time and enjoy the journey.

The Amazing Power of Goal Setting

Another important step you must take in order to succeed in every area of your life is to identify your goals and put them in writing. Goals left to memory, are goals that easily slip out of mind in the busyness of everyday life and responsibilities. Writing your goals down makes them real, and a constant reminder of the life-changing journey you have decided to travel on.

I know for a fact that the people who write their goals down and read them everyday are the ones who succeed.

Be clear when writing your goals. If you want to lose weight don't just write I want to lose weight. Write within 4 weeks I will lose 7 lbs. of fat. Be specific and positive in your goal writing. Make sure your write your goals down, when left to memory goals can easily be forgotten or pushed aside. Reading your goals daily will keep you focused on the action steps you must take in order to make them a reality.

The more you read them and believe the more powerful they become. Post them where you can easily see them. Post a motivational picture or quote that inspires you right next to your goals. Feel them, see them, be them and you will achieve them. Can you feel the excitement of what you are about to accomplish?

I can!

Be as specific as you can on your goal setting. Make sure those goals are realistic and put pressure on yourself by writing deadlines for each one. As you reach your daily and weekly goals you will be building the foundation that will enable you to reach long-term goals. Remember to read your goals everyday for continued inspiration and focus.

I am going to share with you the goals I wrote down over 8 years ago when I first started on my health and fitness journey. If you remember my background, I never played a sport in my life and did not know I was athletic until I started my transformation journey late in life.

My Why's

- Feeling and looking my absolute best

- Wearing a 2 piece and feeling great

- To finally finish something I start

- To have more confidence in myself

- For my father

My Goals

- Within 12 weeks I will gain 7 lbs. of muscle

- Within 12 weeks I will lose 10 lbs. of fat

- I will follow the eating plan

- Within 12 weeks I will have toned abs

- Within 12 weeks I will help 2 people to get in shape

3 Old Negative Thought Patterns

1. Having self defeating/negative thoughts

2. Skipping workouts

3. Not setting goals

New Positive Thought Patterns

1. Picturing myself every day with a strong lean body

2. Go to every workout and give it my all

3. Set goals and follow through

WOW I am actually a little teary reading my first goal sheet. It was written at a time when my confidence was very low and I did not feel good about myself at all. I had just started my transformation journey.

Write down 3 to 4 goals that you would like to work on achieving and write them down in the Hot and Healthy Nutrition and Fitness Journal. Read them daily; post them where you will see it.

When I wrote those goals, I never dreamed that I would accomplish all of them. They seemed so far away and hard to reach. But with a plan, consistency, visualization, time and most important the belief that I could do it, I have reached them and have never looked back.

Your goals may be different than mine. Maybe to fit into a pair of jeans by a certain date, run a 5K by your birthday, kick the sugar habit. There is no right or wrong, just write them down and read them.

Creating A Vision Board

Have you made a Vision Board yet? A vision board is a visual motivator. A Vision board is photos of things you want to manifest in your life such as a fit body, a new home, a place you want to travel to or a charity or cause that you want to be a part of. There is no right or wrong on a vision board. It is something you see every day that inspires you to keep reaching toward your goals.

Once you write down your goals and make a vision board you are putting the wheels in motion for things to happen. Guess what happens when you share your goals with people? They really start to move forward quickly. Watch out, you may just get what you have been dreaming of.

Watch the video at: http://www.youtube.com/watch?v=Vp8S_02f7fY

The Power to Believe Pledge

The power to believe pledge is about signing a contract with your-self. It states you are willing to do what it takes for the next 30 days to follow through with what you start.

I have all I need already within me to change. I have the power to take control of my relationship with food and exercise and the old self-sabotaging beliefs that I have been carrying with me. I am no longer living in the past but living for today and my future.

I believe I can and will reach my health and fitness goals, and I will not be stopped by slow weight loss, plateaus, negative thoughts or feelings, or day to day happenings in life.

Every day I will write in my Hot and Healthy journal; my goals, daily nutrition and my thoughts and feelings and take the time to visualize my goals. I will attach positive motivational photos that make me feel good. I know having a plan of action and being consistent will lead to success.

I understand that this will be a journey, a journey of change and a new way of thinking. There will be ups and downs and I promise to be consistent, patient and persistent.

I am willing to put in the time and effort to get the lasting life long results I truly desire and am meant to have.

I am worth it; my family is worth it and I BELIEVE in myself.

_____   Signature

_____   Date

Your Hot and Healthy Nutrition & Fitness Journal

The Hot and Healthy Nutrition and Fitness Journal is one of the most important tools to use. This is where you are going to write down your goals, journal your nutrition, thoughts and feelings and to be accountable for your fitness workouts.

1. Choose two motivational photos of yourself to put in your Hot and Healthy journal. These pictures should be photos of you that you love and make you happy. Maybe it is a photo of you from childhood or a photo of you with your family. The point is that it should inspire you and make you smile.

2. Write down your WHY in your Hot and Healthy Journal. Take your time doing this step. You may want to think about it, write a little, take a break and then come back to it the next day. Really be with yourself and discover what it is you truly want to get out of this program. Doing this one action step is KEY to your success, so do not skip it. Take your time with it and set the foundation for the program.

3. Next add your goals to the goal pages in the journal. Really take some time with these and think about what it is that you truly want and WHY. Finding your why the real reason you want to get in shape, will make a huge difference in your results. So grab a

cup of green tea and think about your goals before you write them down.

I want you to read your goals EVERYDAY. If you want make a copy of them and stick them on your bathroom mirror, your office at work, on your fridge. The more you see and read them the more you will reach them.

4. In Hot and Healthy Nutrition and Fitness Journal you will find 30 days worth of pages for you to journal your daily nutrition, thoughts and feelings. This is a super important exercise. It will take a few days to get used to writing everything down. Once you get the hang of it you will look forward to keeping track of your nutrition. It will teach you a lot about yourself and what you are really putting in your body. Be honest with yourself and write it down. I don't care if it is a green smoothie or a whole pizza. Just write it down.

Journal how you are feeling that day, what exercise you did. Notice any small changes going on in your body. Are you tired, motivated, hungry, happy, sad? You are encouraged to write anything you want on your journal pages. They are for you and will be a great help to look back at as the weeks go on and see where you have come from and how things are moving along. You might notice a pattern you never realized before or have an AHA moment that pushes you forward. So go journal and see what happens.

What I want you to notice is how you feel, how your body is changing from the inside out. The first thing you will notice when you start an exercise program is that you gain strength, then the body starts to change by losing weight and burning fat and then putting on muscle. Areas of the body will start to become tighter and your clothing will start to become looser.

5. I want you to step on the scale once a week and that is it. The scale is only a guide and one weight loss tool. It can play mind games with us if we let it. Weigh yourself on the same scale, at the same time of day in the morning and write down your weight.

Due to hormone fluctuations, water retention, chemicals in our foods and stress, the scale can go up and down anywhere from about 1 to 5 lbs. in a day. Keep that in mind and notice how you feel, rather than what the scale is saying before you freak out.

Our goal is to trade fat for muscle and muscle weighs more than fat. We are working for sexy curvy muscle in this program, not bodybuilding muscle so relax.

Keep moving forward and don't stop. If you fall off the wagon, accept it and move on. It is OK. We all fall off. There really is no wagon, and it's the people who get right back at the next meal that are successful.

6. In the Hot and Healthy Nutrition and Fitness Journal use your "Success Calendar". Each day that you complete your workout, mark a big X in your favorite colored magic marker on that day. This is a great visual reminder and motivator. When you start seeing all the days crossed off you know you are well on your way.

7. Look over the exercise circuits in the program and get familiar with them. You will be doing one new circuit each week.

8. Look at the 7-Day Meal plan sample ideas in the journal. I have given you 7 days of easy clean eating ideas. Use these as guidelines on how to plan your meals for the next thirty days. If you are vegetarian or vegan then replace the protein sources with other options from the shopping list that meet your dietary needs.

There really are no fancy recipes in the first 30 days. The easier the better and you will stick to it in the first 30 days. Mix and match or make up your own meals. Just follow the guidelines. You will find more ideas on my web site www.LauraLondonFitness.com After the 30 days you will start to incorporate new recipes and combinations.

Have you ever sat down and made your own weekly meal plan? Are you wishing I had given you 30 days of what to eat? There is a reason I did not. I want you to be in charge, I want you to understand once and for all what putting together healthy meals is all about. If I do it all for you you will never fully learn. We learn by doing. So I am giving you a sample and want you to create your own meals with the foods you like and will eat. Not the foods I like. We are all different and have different tastes. Some of you may eat meat and some of you may be vegetarian but the principals are still the same.

There is a great web site called www.PepperPlate.com that you can use. Collect the recipes you like and print out your own meal plans with recipes you find on my web site and on the internet. I highly suggest you check it out.

You have all you need within you for success; I am just here to help guide you along the way!

Hot & Healthy Nutrition 101

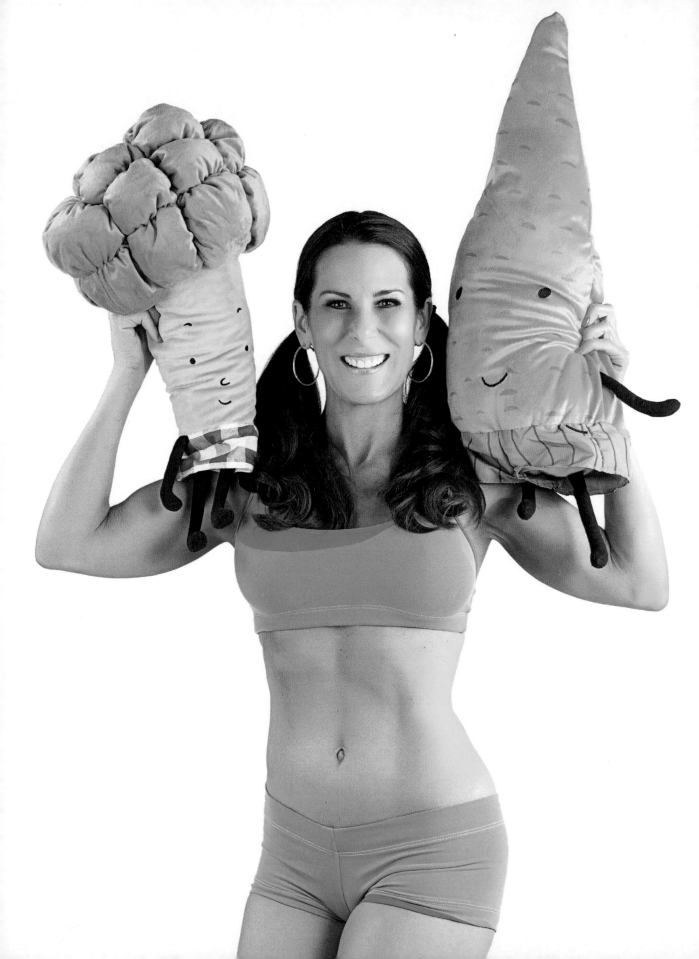

Hot & Healthy Nutrition Made Easy

Eating should not be so crazy and confusing. What happened to the days when we ate to enjoy and to be healthy? We have almost come to the point where women don't even know how to feed themselves any more. Prepackaged diet food is becoming a way of life for a lot of women and their families.

Life is busy and convenience food is easy to buy, easy to take with you and easy to feed to the children. But wait, stop, hold everything. Have you read the labels of the packaged food? Seriously, when did we lose our ability to read? To comprehend the written word?

We know deep down that the more natural a food is the better it is for our body, right? We know we should be eating more "Foods From Mother Nature". But the question to answer is WHY? Why are we not doing it?

I believe the reason is that we have gotten bombarded by so much misinformation, we have become confused, and mainly we are tired, frustrated, and have just plain given up on trying to eat healthy.

Eating healthy can really be very simple if you apply the principles I am going to share with you. They are the foundations of how I live my life and eat everyday.

I have made it simple for you, going back to the basics. You are going to enjoy eating again, eating real food and feeding real food to your family.

You are going to get excited when the weight starts coming off, when you are not tired any more, when the crazy hormonal outburst of emotions fade away, when your complexion clears up and when you just feel good everyday when you get out of bed.

You need to eat to lose weight, period end of story. So lets talk about how much to eat and when to eat. My main goal here is to get you to eat consistently throughout the day and understand what portion sizes you should be eating to reach your goal weight. I don't want your main focus to be about calorie counting but I do want you to realize what and how much you are eating.

Lets talk about your Basal Metabolic Rate or BMR. This is how many calories you burn if you just sit and do nothing all day. It's the amount of calories your body uses every day just to keep you alive. Here is the formula to find your BMR. This is the minimum amount of calories you need a day to not send your body into starvation mode.

655 + (4.35 x your weight in pounds) + 4.7 x (height in inches) – 4.7 (ages in years)

You can also use a BMR calculator at: http://www.bmi-calculator. net/bmr-calculator/

I am 5' 3", weight 115 and am 47. The bare minimum amount of calories for me to eat would be 1230 a day. This is if I did nothing all day long, but sit on the couch. The reason for me showing you this is so you do not eat too little (like so many woman do) and get frustrated because you are not losing weight. Remember, you need to eat to lose weight!

This is how I want you to eat for the next 30 days (and more). It will become second nature and then it will be easy to stick you your nutrition plan. Eating in this calorie range, especially on the days you exercise will keep your metabolism running like a racecar in the Indy 500. Don't let it hit the wall by not eating enough. Set a timer on your phone if you need to remind yourself to eat.

Guidelines

Time	Meal	Calories
7:00 AM	Breakfast	400
10:00 AM	Snack	150 - 200
1:00 PM	Lunch	400
3:00 PM	Snack	150 - 200
6 - 7 PM	Dinner	400
Total Calories		1500 - 1600

Do not skip meals! It will wreak havoc for the rest of the day.

Breakfast or before a workout – I want you to eat breakfast. If you are one of those people who just can't stomach breakfast or are working out early in the morning and can't eat a lot, then just start with something small. Try a protein shake or 1/2 a small banana or piece of fruit. Do not do this eat 1/2 banana workout out and then not eat until lunch. This is not enough food to fuel your body.

Eating After a workout – There is a wonderful window of opportunity to eat after your workout. Your body is ready and begging for fuel. Eat within a 30-60 minute window after working out. Eat a meal that has both protein and carbs to refuel yourself, help repair damaged muscles, and replenish your glycogen stores. It could be a protein shake, green smoothie, eggs and oatmeal, a healthy protein muffin or maybe nuts and a nice juicy orange. There are so many combinations you can come up with.

A Note on Proteins, Carbs & Fats

Proteins

- Protein has 4 calories per gram

- Protein takes extra energy to digest, up to 1 calorie per gram

- Protein is essential for muscle growth

- Protein takes up to 3 hours to digest

Carbohydrates

- Carbs have 4 calories per gram

- Two types Simple & Complex

- Easily converted into energy & easily converted into body fat

- Takes 10 minutes and up to 2 hours to be digested

Fats

- Fats have 9 calories per gram

- Fats are essential for proper brain, body function

- Fats are essential for balanced hormones

- They take up to 4 hours to be digested

- You need good fats in your diet to lose weight

"When you feel like you again there will be no stopping you in any area of your life. Because when you feel good about yourself there is nothing you can't do or achieve."

~Laura London~

Let's Talk Healthy Eating

Healthy eating is about eating a diet rich in whole foods and avoiding processed foods. Healthy eating will help you lose weight but even more important than weight loss is becoming the healthiest version of you.

We are going to be nourishing the body with real nutrient dense foods. We will also learn about alkalizing the body, balancing our blood sugar and eating consistency throughout the day.

The Pillars of Healthy Eating

1. Eat organic fruits and vegetables. Fruits and veggies are filled with complex carbohydrates, fiber, protein and vitamin and minerals. Eating a lot of veggies will fill you up with few calories. Fruit is great, and supplies the body with vitamins and minerals but it also has a lot of sugar. Excess carbohydrates will add fat to the body.

2. Keep a healthy balance between carbs and protein. Try to have some protein with each meal. Protein will help to keep you satisfied longer and balance your blood sugar. Protein can come from organic meat, organic dairy, GMO free tofu, veggies, nuts and legumes. Choose 100% whole grains. Remember veggies are complex carbs and are excellent choices over rice, pasta and potatoes. Try quinoa, millet, brown rice and sprouted breads.

Organic and grass fed meats should always be your first choice. Non-organic meats can be filled with hormones and drugs, which can interfere with your body's delicate hormones and metabolic function. Which in turn can possibly interfere with your body's ability to lose weight. Trust me it is worth the extra money and your body will thank you.

3. Cut out all processed foods. Your body does not know what to do with processed foods and they turn the body acidic. When the body is acidic disease can take hold. Again they are hormone disruptors and can lead to a malfunctioning thyroid and a burned out metabolism. GET RID OF THEM NOW.

4. Journal your food for 30 days. I am super serious about this. Write down everything you eat for the next 30 days. EVERYTHING. It is a documented fact that people who journal their food will be more successful at weight loss. Write it down every meal, every day. TAKE RESPONSIBILITY no matter what you eat, good or bad, and write it in your food journal.

5. Don't be afraid of good healthy fats. The brain is made up of 90% fat. The body needs the correct fats to run efficiently. Fats will keep you fuller longer. Did you know that eating the correct types of fats would help you lose fat! Some good fats include, raw coconut oil, olive oil, nuts, avocados, and flax seed.

6. Eat during the day. Some of us do better eating 4-5 times a day, and others do great with eating 3 larger meals a day. Do what works best for you and your body type. The point is that you need to eat and eat good quality food to lose weight.

7. Do not skip meals – Planning is KEY in being successful. Plan out your meals for a day or even a week in advance. Always have a healthy snack in your purse or car so you don't get caught skipping a meal and then binging because you are starving.

8. Water – Drink up to 1/2 your body weight in water. Most people, especially women don't get enough water. Water will help to detox the body, hydrate your skin and reduce belly bloating. Our goal is to drink up to ½ our body weight in water. Some days we will and some days we won't and that is OK. The foods we are going to be eating are going to be high water content foods so you will be sure you are getting enough water on the Hot and Healthy Body Plan. Drinking ice cold water has been shown to burn more calories than drinking room temperature water.

How much should you drink? Drink up to 1/2 your body weight in ounces of water. If you weigh 150 lbs. drink up to 75 ounces daily.

I add lemon or orange slices to my water. Essential oils are great to add to your water too. Have you ever tried peppermint water? It's delicious and refreshing. I drink what I call my "Workout Water" everyday, water with one drop of **peppermint oil** and 3 drops of **lemon oil**. Love it!

"WATER - Did you know that if your body is mildly dehydrated it could shut down fat burning and raise cortisol levels. CORTISOL is the FAT STORAGE hormone"

9. Alcohol – Skip it for 30 days. I would prefer none for the first 30 days. Alcohol is full of empty calories; it slows down your fat burning and causes dehydration. When you are drinking you are more likely to splurge on high calorie foods and get off track. If you absolutely have to, then please limit yourself to no more than 2 drinks a week.

10. Kick Soy to the curb. I am not a big fan of soy. It is highly processed and frequently genetically modified (GMO). Those veggie burgers in the grocery store can be loaded with GMO, salt and are what I consider a processed food or FRANKENFOOD. Soy can also interfere with your thyroid function, which can equal weight loss nightmares.

I am not saying not to eat soy, just realize the type and how much of it you are eating. If you are going to eat soy make sure it is organic and non-GMO, and in it's most natural form. I prefer the large white blocks of tofu that you find soaked in water. Organic Nam Shoyu is an unpasteurized soy sauce and adds nice flavor to food. I would suggest limiting the amount of soy you eat.

11. Coffee, Tea & Soda. No more than 2 cups per day of coffee or caffeinated tea. Too much caffeine over stimulates your adrenal system and can contribute to adrenal fatigue, restless sleep and wreck havoc on your endocrine system.

Some great alternatives are Teeccino, caffeine-free herbal coffee or Dandelion coffee. Try Matcha organic green tea one of nature's natural fat burners. I like DoMatcha Green Tea. One cup of Matcha Green Tea has 137 times the amount of antioxidants compared to 1 cup of green tea. WOW!

Another one of my favorites for natural fat burning help is Oolong tea. It has a high concentration of the antioxidant polyphenol, which helps block fat-building enzymes.

Soda and high calorie drinks. Do I even have to go over this? Get rid of them. That is all I am going to say. If you have to have bubbly, a great alternative is sparkling water, such as LA Croix or Perrier. Add in a packet of Emergen-C or E-Boost for a low calorie low sugar pop of natural flavor. It's great and will satisfy your soda craving.

12. Use Celtic sea salt. Please get rid of table salt. It is highly processed and again not natural. The body needs natural salts to function properly. Natural Sea Salts are loaded with over 90 trace minerals that your body needs and uses. So feel free to add a sprinkle of natural salt to your foods if you like.

13. No artificial sweeteners. You know what I am talking about, the little blue and pink packets. They are in my opinion highly toxic. From now on think of them as little packets of rat poison. "A little RAT POISON with your coffee today, sweetie?"

Artificial sweeteners are a FRANKENFOOD and your body does not know what to do with it or how to process it. Do you know where your body will store these highly toxic chemical sweeteners? In your fat cells! It is trying to protect your vital organs and get it as far away from them as possible. I cringe every time I see people reaching for those colored packets, I want to scream, "Stop. Put that back!"

Stevia, honey, agave, and natural sweeteners are OK in moderation. I would even prefer natural sugar to an artificial sweetener. A teaspoon of natural sugar has only 15 calories. You can find stevia in powdered or liquid form.

14. How much protein? This is a big question with a lot of different answers. Protein aids in fat loss and building lean muscle mass, regulates blood sugar and aids in muscle recovery. The suggested amount is anywhere from .6 to .8 grams of protein for every pound of body weight. So if you weigh 150 lbs. your range would be 90 to 120 grams of protein a day.

If you are a meat eater then this is easy to do. If you are vegetarian or vegan you can still easily get all the protein you need from plants, nuts and seeds.

Most important is to listen to your body. There is no right or wrong, meaning you don't have to get 120 grams of protein in every single day. We are not going for a bodybuilding contest here. We are going for a healthy body. Trust me your muscles will not fall off if you do not eat protein at every single meal for the rest of your life. I find if people relax a little and enjoy eating more, their weight falls off faster.

15. Green Drinks/Juicing/Green Smoothies. I am a huge fan of juicing, green smoothies and green drinks. Make sure your green smoothies are not loaded with sugar from fruit. Adding any of these options into your nutrition plan will help to cut your cravings down. Yes, you heard me right. They are full of nutrition and when your body is nutritionally satisfied you will not have those crazy cravings, especially ones for sugar. SUGAR IS EVIL.

If you like to juice, make sure you are using more veggies than fruit in your juices. I have a great juicing book which you can find on www.7DayGoddessJuiceFeast.com with over 30 recipes in it. It is a great place to start if you are new to juicing.

Green drinks are basically green foods in a powder form that you add to water. They are highly nutritious, easy to use and pack a powerful punch of vitamin and minerals to your diet.

16. Getting Enough Sleep. You're a woman and generally we do not stop going all day long. Are you getting enough sleep? I cannot stress the importance of getting enough sleep. You need a good seven to nine hours of restful sleep a night. When you sleep your body has a chance to repair, detox and rebuild. Insufficient sleep can cause your growth hormone level to decrease, which can increase your chances for gaining weight!

Just like you are scheduling your exercises I want you to schedule enough time to sleep. Your body will thank you for it. **Lavender essential oil** is a great item to have on your nightstand. It helps to relax and calm the body, will help you destress from the day and to have a restful night of sleep. Want to sleep like a baby? Put a drop on your hands and breathe in then place a drop on your pillow. Night-night.

"Hot and Healthy REWARD MEALS"

It is just about impossible to eat "perfect" 100% of the time. People can do it for a few weeks or even a few months, but then guess what? It ultimately back fires. Think of all the times people go on diets for a special occasion. When that special occasion has come and gone they go back to their old eating habits and put the weight right back on. This is called the Yo-Yo effect or rebound effect.

Follow the Hot and Healthy guidelines 90% of the time. The other 10%, eat for pure enjoyment.

100% nutritional discipline is never really needed to completely change your body. And that extra 10% means you can feel free to eat the food you love.

So "The Hot and Healthy" way is to give you a simple instruction: eat any food you like, in up to 10% of your meals; in the other 90% of your meals, eat the foods that will fuel your body with high quality nutrition for success. That ratio will give you the body you want AND allow you to enjoy the food you love. I truly believe that once you tell yourself you can't have a food you love you have just set yourself up to fail. The Hot and Healthy way is to never deny yourself of anything. But hold on; make sure you do the math. Let's find out what that 10% really is. Make sure you do the math and determine what 10% of the time really means.

For example, if you're eating 5 meals per day for 7 days of the week – that's 35 meals. 10% of 35 meals are about 3.5 meals. Therefore you're allowed to enjoy your "Hot and Healthy REWARD Meals" on 3 meals each week. If you skip a meal or eat something not on the plan, that counts as a Hot and Healthy Reward Meal. Remember this is not for life but for 30 days. You can do this for 30 days and guess what? After 30 days you are going to be so successful you are going to want to keep going.

Make sure your 10% doesn't become 20% or 30%. This does not mean you can go crazy and eat a whole gallon of ice cream, half a pizza or spend the whole day eating whatever you want. Oh no, quite the opposite. Just like you plan your exercise days, I want you to plan your reward meals.

Rather, into your diet and can enjoy your 10% "Hot and Healthy Reward Meal" should include some foods, in reasonable quantities, that might not normally fit into your plan. This might be a slice of pizza or an appetizer and a glass of wine with dinner. For me it is anything chocolate.

One way to prevent "overdoing it" is to schedule your 10% meals. This way you know when and what you will be adding into your diet and can enjoy you 10% with no guilt knowing you deserve it.

What Does A Serving Size Look Like?

Easy Guidelines for portion sizes. These are just guidelines to make eating a little easier when you are planning a meal or dining out. Portion size varies for everyone.

What is a serving? Here are some guidelines to follow to make it easier.

Protein, Palm Size - 15-30 grams 1 chicken breast,

Carb, Fist Size - about 15 - 20 grams a serving or 1/2 cup or 1 piece of fruit

Fat, Size of a dime - 10 -15 grams per serving. 20-30 Fat grams a day (About 2-3 Servings)

Greens - 5 servings or more

Water up to 1/2 your body weight in ounces

Once you have these guides in your head, the combinations you can come up with are endless. Again, eating should be easy, eating should nourish the body and eating should be simple and a pleasure.

Protein & Carb Portion Sizes

Per Meal Eating 4-5 Times A Day

If you weigh:

Under 120 lbs. = about 15-20 gram portion sizes

Example 15 grams Carb & 15 Grams Protein

120-135 lbs. = about 20-25 gram portion sizes

Example 20 grams Carb & 20 Grams Protein

Over 136 lbs. = about 25-30 gram portion sizes

Example 25 grams Carb & 25 Grams Protein

Set yourself up for success and to save time if you can buy food items in portion controlled containers, especially if you have a hard time with portion control.

Cook in advance and make large portions for the rest of the week. Make a crock pot of chili or large soup and put in individual containers and freeze. Try making a large salad, put just a small amount of dressing on it and keep in fridge, it will last for up to 5 days and again you can grab and go. I also make a pan of roasted veggies at the beginning of the week and have them to throw into salad and wraps or as a side dish all week long.

Think plan, prepare and eat.

Examples:

- 6 oz. Organic Greek Yogurt Containers

- Small Bag of Carrots

- Green Smoothie

- Hummus Containers

- Organic Cheese sticks

- Free Range Hard Boiled Eggs

- Natural Protein Bars

- Make your own small bags of nuts (2 oz.)

Fruit is Naturally Portion Sized

You can take your favorite healthy food and put it in portion-sized containers so you can GRAB & GO.

Sugar = Carbohydrates Carbohydrates = Sugar

The body only needs a certain amount of carbohydrates/sugar a day and anything more than that it will store as fat on our bodies. The best way I have found to reduce body fat is to monitor the amount of carbohydrates/sugar you eat a day. I am not saying to cut carbs out of your diet, not at all. I don't believe in cutting any food group out. But monitoring the amount of carbs/sugar you eat in a day can have a significant affect on your weight loss.

The body naturally only has 1 tsp. of glucose (sugar) in it's blood stream at a time. It works very hard to keep this tight ratio. When you eat too many carbs/sugar the body will take the extra sugar out of your blood and store it in fat cells to protect the body, especially if you are not exercising.

If you have a greater quantity of carbohydrates entering the body than can be used immediately for energy or stored in the form of glycogen (which the body stores in very small amounts), the excess is rapidly converted into triglycerides and stored in the form of body fat.

Each 5 grams (20 calories) of carbohydrates is approximately the equivalent of one teaspoon of sugar. Start checking your food labels and see how much sugar you are really eating a day. The average person eats 60-70 teaspoons of sugar a day. If this sugar was kept in your system, your health would be jeopardized, so the body tries to protect itself by converting the excess sugar to stored body fat.

All carbohydrates are broken down to sugar in the body. So keep in mind that even 100% whole grains and quality complex carbs like brown rice, quinoa or sweet potatoes still break down as sugar in the body. I will teach you about carbohydrates and the glycemic index later in the Hot and Healthy book. The main point I want you to understand here is that even if you are eating better quality carbs say brown rice vs. candy they both break down into sugar in the body. One form just does it a little faster than the other.

What to Look For in the Grocery Story

Organic

- 100% whole grain

- Hormone & Antibiotic Free

- Toxic Free

- Chemical Free

- Non GMO

Stay Away from:

- High Fructose Corn Syrup

- White Sugar

- White Flour

- Genetically Modified Foods

- Artificial Sweeteners

- Sugar Free

- Artificially colored or flavored

- Packaged "Frankenfoods"

- Excessive sodium

- Deli Meats with Nitrates

- Fruit Juices, too much sugar

- Too Many Dried Fruits

Laura London Approved Shopping List

Proteins	Dairy / Eggs
Organic Chicken Breast	Fat Free Organic Greek Yoghurt
Lean Ground Chicken or Turkey	Organic Cottage Cheese 1%
Turkey Bacon (Nitrate Free)	Unsweetened Almond, Coconut, Rice, Hemp, Milk
Pork Chops	Organic Grass Fed Butter
Filet Mignon	Organic Eggs or Liquid Egg Whites
Grass Fed Lean Beef	String Cheese
Sirloin Steak	Feta, Parmesan, Gorgonzola
Bison	Keifer
Seafood	Vegetarian Protein
Salmon	Tofu
Tilapia	Seitan
Flounder	Tempeh
Sole	TVP (Texturized Veggie Protein)
Cod	Vegan Protein Powders
Tuna - Tuna Fish	
Mahi Mahi	
Scallops	
Shrimp	
Crab Meat	

Starchy Carbs	Complex Carbs - Fruit
Old Fashioned & Steel Cut Oats	Berries, Strawberries, Blueberries, Raspberries, Goji Berries
Brown Rice	Lemon & Limes
Quinoa, Millet, Amaranth, Farro, Buckwheat	Apples
100% Whole Grain Pasta	Orange
Organic Brown Rice Cakes	Pear
Sprouted Grain Breads, Wraps	Banana (Limit 1 per day)
100% Whole Wheat Bread, Tortillas	Watermelon
Brown Rice Bread, Wraps	Honey Dew
Ryvita & Mary's Gone Crackers	Cantaloupe
Sweet Potato	Grapefruit
Couscous	Kiwi
Beans / Legumes	Pineapple
Black beans, kidney beans, garbanzo beans, etc.	Peach
Lentils	Nectarine

Veggies	Oils & Fats
Asparagus	Olive Oil (First cold pressed is always best)
Broccoli	Raw Coconut oil, flax, walnut, almond etc. (First cold pressed is always best
Spinach	Flax seeds, Chia seeds, Hemp seeds, Savi seeds
Zucchini	Nut Butters (in moderation)
Cauliflower	Butter (Grass Fed)
Eggplant	Nuts & Seeds
Green Beans	Try different flavored oils to dress up your cooking. They come in a variety of flavors.
Artichokes	
Brussel Sprouts	
Lettuce, aragula, romaine, bib, butter, etc.	
Sprouts	
Kale	
Carrots	
Tomato	
Mushrooms	
Celery	
Onions	
Cucumbers	
Peppers	
Edamame	
Avocado	

Spices & Condiments
All fresh & dried spices
Stevia
Cinnamon (my favorite)
Salsa (low sodium)
Mustard
Ketchup (No High Fructose Corn Syrup)
100% Natural Jam
Low Fat Natural Salad Dressing
Balsamic Vinegar, Flavored Vinegars (these are great)
Tamari/Nama Shoyu
Low Sodium Organic Chicken or Veggie Broth
Fruit Zest
Vanilla & Natural Extracts
Maca
Organic Dark Chocolate
Raw Cacao nibs and powder
Braggs Liquid Aminos & Coconut Aminos

7 Day Hot & Healthy Meal Ideas

I have planned out 7 days of basic and easy meal ideas as a guide. I wanted to give you examples of meal idea combinations that fit the Hot and Healthy Nutrition Program.

Again, this is not about calorie counting or depravation. It is about learning how to eat again and enjoy your food while loosing weight at the same time.

I encourage you to branch out and experiment with new recipes and combinations. Don't worry a cook book is in the works with lots of healthy meal ideas.

Follow the guidelines, eat consistently throughout the day and make sure to get in your cardio and weight training workouts.

Remember: DIET's don't work; they are only a temporary solution. When you reach your goal weight by eating healthy natural foods, you can start to include a few more starchy carbs. You will know if you start gaining weight, that you will need to reduce the carbs and exercise a little more.

Once you have reached your goal weight, always strive to stay within 5 lbs. of your goal weight. You worked hard to get there now keep it there for life.

Day One

Start Each Day with a glass of water with fresh squeezed lemon juice.

Breakfast

1 Piece of Fruit
4 egg whites & 1 Yolk
Unlimited Veggies, spinach, peppers
1-cup decaf green tea

Snack

Fat Free Greek Yogurt with fresh fruit

Or

Green Smoothie, Almond Milk or water, protein powder, spinach, frozen strawberries or blueberries

Lunch

4 oz. chicken breast (grilled or baked)
1-2 cups favorite veggies steamed or large green salad w veggies ½ cup brown rice, or sweet potato
Oil & Vinegar w lemon juice or low fat natural dressing

Snack

3-4 oz. of hummus with 1 cups raw veggies

Dinner

4 oz. fish or chicken (salmon, tuna, halibut, etc.)
Unlimited steamed veggies, fresh squeezed garlic &
Lemon juice, olive oil

Day Two

Start Each Day with a glass of water with fresh squeezed lemon juice.

Breakfast

4 egg white omelet (1 Yolk is fine) with veggies
½ cup oatmeal or 1-2 slice Ezekiel Bread
1 tsp. raw coconut oil or 1 tbsp. 100% jam

Snack

1 med apple
10 almonds (unsalted)
Protein Shake

Lunch

¾ cup black beans or 4 oz. chicken breast, on salad loaded with
veggies (for example-tomatoes, baby spinach, peppers, cucumbers,
shredded carrots, mushrooms,
1 orange or apple

Snack

½ bell pepper sliced, 10 cherry tomatoes, ½ cucumber
3-4 oz. nitrate free turkey slices & piece of fruit

Or

Protein Shake with blueberries, strawberries ½ frozen banana, ½ Cucumber
8 – 10 oz. water or almond milk

Dinner

4- 5 oz. Flank steak or chicken seasoned w garlic & spices
Unlimited steamed or grilled veggies

Day Three

Start Each Day with a glass of water with fresh squeezed lemon juice.

Breakfast

Berry smoothie - 1 scoop vanilla protein powder, 1 cup frozen berries of choice, 1/2 banana.

Snack

Plain Greek Yoghurt, Chopped Apple & a few raisins, Crushed Almonds, Chia Seeds, Cinnamon, Stevia to taste.

Lunch

4 oz. grilled chicken or lean turkey burger
1 small sweet potato
1 cup of your favorite green veggies steamed or raw

Snack

1/4 cup White bean dip or hummus w. raw veggies

Or

Guacamole with veggies

Or

1 oz. Organic Cheese w. 1 orange or apple

Dinner

4 oz. of chicken, fish, egg whites, or beans
Spring mix salad w. lots of different veggies, balsamic vinegar or Natural Low Fat Salad Dressing

Day Four

Start Each Day with a glass of water with fresh squeezed lemon juice.

Breakfast

4 egg whites + 1 yolk scrambled with salsa top
1/2 cup oatmeal or 1-2 slices Ezekiel Toast or
1 grapefruit with stevia or 1/2 cantaloupe

Snack

1/2 Cup cottage cheese or Greek Yoghurt
1 cup mixed berries or fresh fruit

Lunch

Teriyaki Grilled Chicken with lettuce wraps
Tomatoes, lettuce, sprouts, salsa, hot sauce

Snack

1 apple with 2 tbsp. almond butter

Or

Protein Bar

Or

Green Smoothie

Dinner

4 oz. of a lean protein of your choice
Asparagus, with garlic, soy sauce and olive oil

Day Five

Start Each Day with a glass of water with fresh squeezed lemon juice.

Breakfast

Green Smoothie, water or almond milk, protein powder, veggies, berries, flax, bee pollen, 1/2 cucumber.

Oatmeal pancake, 4 whites, 1 yolk, 1/2 cup oatmeal, cinnamon. Blend in a blender and cook in pan. Top with 100% fruit jam.

Snack

2 celery stalk / baby carrots with 1 tbsp. almond butter in each.
2 hard-boiled eggs

Lunch

Tuna Fish on a bed of baby greens with mixed veggies
1 Apple

Snack

1/4 cup of hummus and 1-cup raw veggies

Or

Protein shake w. piece of fruit

Dinner

Turkey burger on a grilled portabella mushroom.
Spring mix salad with your choice of veggies.
Olive oil & vinegar dressing, lemon juice or balsamic vinegar.

Day Six

Start Each Day with a glass of water with fresh squeezed lemon juice.

Breakfast

Breakfast burrito - 2 corns or 1 gluten-free tortilla
Scrambled 4 egg whites w/tomatoes, onions, bell peppers or salsa.
Green tea.

Snack

Greek Yoghurt, topped with cinnamon, stevia, mixed berries, sprinkle of oatmeal, raw wheat germ or Kashi Go Lean

Lunch

Grilled Chicken on green spring mix salad or spinach, 10 cherry tomatoes, cucumber slices, olive oil, vinegar.

Steamed Broccoli.

Snack

Protein Shake & Vita muffin

Or

1 Apple & 10 Almonds

Dinner

4 oz. beans (your favorite- black, pinto, chick peas, etc.)
Or 5 oz. lean protein: chicken, fish, shrimp with spices.
1 cup of veggies steamed, grilled or in a salad with olive/vinegar dressing.

Day Seven

Start Each Day with a glass of water with fresh squeezed lemon juice.

Breakfast

French Toast 1 to 2 slices of 100% whole grain bread, or Ezekiel, 4 egg whites, cinnamon, and vanilla extract for batter, can use protein powder too. Top with your favorite fruit - apple slices of fresh berries.

Snack

1 med pear or piece of fruit of your choice (try frozen grapes, yum!)
15 almonds.

Lunch

5 oz. Grilled chicken chopped.
Spring mix salad, unlimited veggies.
1 tbsp. dressing.
1/2 brown rice or 1/2 cup Quinoa or 1 small sweet potato.

Snack

Cucumber slices, 15 cherry tomatoes, celery, 1/4 of an avocado.
Your favorite bean or hummus.

Dinner

Marinated Shrimp on a skewer with Grilled Veggies served on a bed of spinach cooked in 1 tbsp. olive oil and garlic.

Laura London's Nutritional Laws

• *Cut out the "Franken Foods" & Artificial Sweeteners*

• *Eat Breakfast Every Morning*

• *Start the Day Off with Water & Fresh Squeezed Lemon Juice*

• *Eat 4-5 Times A Day*

• *Loan up on Veggies, Fruits/Berries and Lean Proteins Every Day*

• *Your Goal For Each Meal is BALANCE*

• *Consume 25-50 Grams of Fiber a Day*

• *Eat Within 1 Hour of Getting Up*

• *Drink Up To 1/2 your Body Weight In Water Each Day*

• *Avoid Refined, Flour, Grains, Diet Soda & Fruit Juices. Don't Drink Your Calories*

• *Try A Vegetarian or Raw Food Day Once a Week*

• *If you Booze You Looze, Alcohol Will Prevent Fat Loss*

• *Limit Carbs in Your Evening Meal*

• *Understand Portion Sizes*

• *Go to Bed a Little Hungry, it's Ok and great for fat burning*

• *Get a Good Night Sleep Each Night*

• *Learn to Awaken Your Foods With Spices*

• *Plan Out Your Meals in Advance and Be Prepared*

Why Use A Protein Powder?

Protein, we all know we need it; we all know it's good for us. But what does protein really do for us? Protein helps to keep hormones balanced; it is good for your skin, nails, hair and metabolism. It is an important component of every cell in your body.

Your body uses protein to build and repair tissue, bones, muscles, cartilage, skin and blood. Boy, protein has a lot of work to do! Protein is known as the building blocks of your body.

The body needs to expend energy (burn calories) to digest protein. Protein has 7 calories per gram. So lets say you just ate a 4 oz. chicken breast that has roughly 110 calories. The body will use energy to digest and process that chicken breast, so the chicken may only be worth about 80 to 90 calories. Pretty cool.

We want to get the best quality protein into our bodies. Some high quality sources of protein are organic hormone free chicken, grass fed beef, organic eggs, wild caught fish and organic vegetables and plant based proteins.

Plant based proteins such as vegetables, and plant protein powders supply the body with nutrients, enzymes and fiber. They are alkalizing to the body and a great way to get protein into the body.

I get a lot of questions about protein powders to supplement the diet with. Protein powders are a great way to add protein to the body quickly and easily.

We don't always have time to cook a chicken breast or make a hummus wrap and take it on the run with us. I love protein shakes and green smoothies as a way to get that muscle building, body repairing, and beautifying protein into the body. They should be in addition to eating real high quality food not in place of food all the time.

Look for high quality protein powders without artificial colors, flavors and highly processed sweeteners.

I have been using Purium Health Products for well over 10 years. The company is green, organic and GMO free certified. This is the how I stay lean and green all year long.

Purium has the healthiest 10 Day Transformation you will ever find. The 10-Day Celebrity Transformation. 90-Day results in just 10 days! Real people, Real results, Real fast, that last a lifetime.

Visit: www.phporder.com/lauralondon

Hot & Healthy Exercise 101

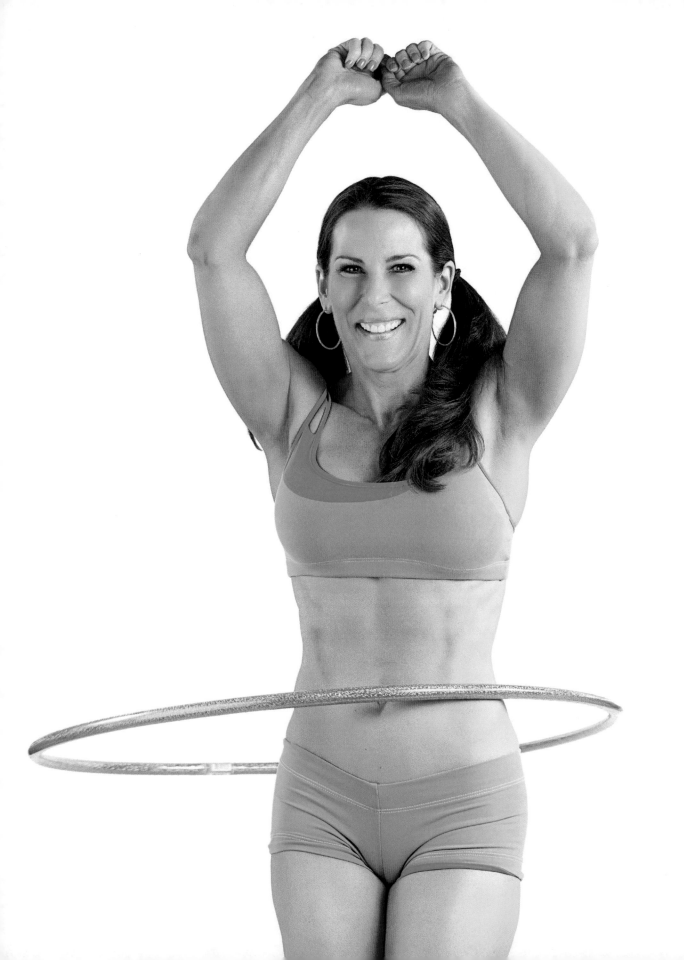

Exercise 101

Well here we are at the fitness portion of the book. So far we have talked about healthy eating and good nutrition. Now we are going to talk about your soon to be amazing Hot and Healthy Body. Now that you have learned the foundations of eating for your health, I want to talk about exercise.

Exercise should be fun and something you look forward to. Remember when we talked about creating a positive mindset in an earlier chapter. Now is the time when I really want you to put that thinking in ACTION.

Each time you get ready to exercise I want you to think of all the beautiful things you are doing for your body such as, lowering cardiac risks, promoting strong healthy bones, improving your digestive and mental health. Increasing your immune system not to mention more restful sleep you can add in better self-confidence. Wow! Just think of all the wonderful things we are doing for ourselves just by exercising! You must really love yourself.

Why do you think up until now it has not been easy to stick to an exercise program? Is it lack of willpower, time, focus, kids, family? We could go on. I believe it is because you have not been truly engaged and in tune with your own body and how it operates.

We are given these miraculous bodies and someone forgot to give us the instruction manual on how they operate most efficiently. Once you have the directions it makes everything so much easier and it all starts to make sense. You will be in control and know how to build your own Hot and Healthy body.

We are not going to spend hours in the gym or on cardio equipment. Are you jumping up and down yet? We are going to work that Goddess Body efficiently to get the most bang for our exercise buck. The Hot and Healthy workout system is based on science and mother nature. What a great combination.

We are going to tap into the "fountain of youth" otherwise known as (HGH) human growth hormone. When you tap into this lovely magical hormone you will be helping to turning back the clock. Tapping into this hormone can improve your muscle mass, fat burning ability and even help you achieve a beautiful goddess glowing complexion while at the same time balancing your hormones. Now I say that is a win-win combination.

Math has never been my "thing" but here is a math equation I think you can relate to that will make you understand the rest of this chapter.

Exercise = More strength = More Muscle = Fat Loss = Hot and Health Body.

Each circuit workout in the Hot and Healthy program is designed to get your heart rate pumping, fire up your fat burning metabolism and tighten and tone every square inch of your amazing body. While at the same time, stimulate your body's natural detox system, your lymph system, at the same time. Talk about total body wellness at its best.

Hot and Healthy Body Exercise Benefits:

- You will burn many more calories during your circuit workout than being on a treadmill for the same amount of time

- You will be using every muscle group to maximize fat burning long after you stop working out

- You will be tapping into your "fountain of youth" hormone for anti-aging benefits

- You will be tightening and toning every square inch of your Goddess Body during each circuit workout

- You will be engaged and having fun while getting fit and fabulous knowing you are in control of your hot and healthy body

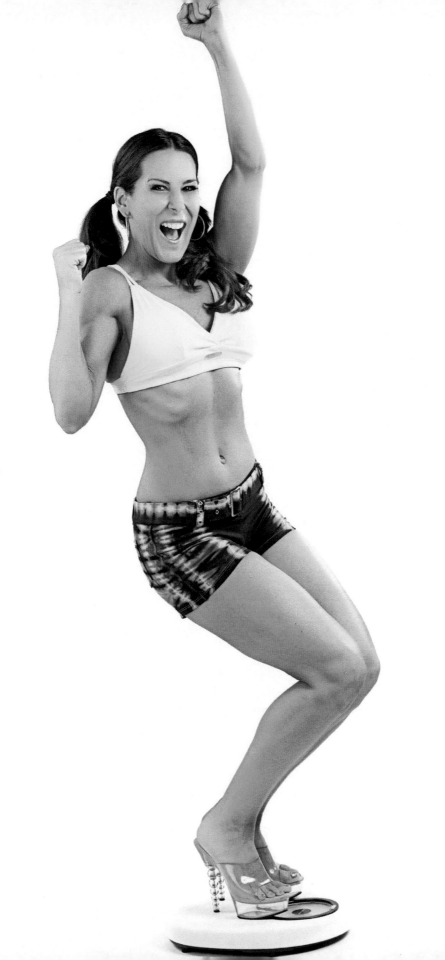

Exercise 101
Week 1

Welcome to week one! Are you ready to get started? I know you are, so here we go. The beauty of the Hot and Healthy exercise program is that anyone can do it. So don't worry if you have not exercised in a long time, I have got you covered. On the other hand, if you are a fitness diva, the Hot and Healthy program is going to work for you, too! How, you ask? Well, let me explain.

If you are just starting out you may want to go through the circuit one time and work on building up your strength and endurance. If you are already working out then run through the circuits two or three times for a heart pumping, fat-burning, muscle-building workout.

Another way to adjust the program is to adjust your intensity, meaning you can move your body slower or faster. Yet another way to adjust the program is to start with no weights and as you progress add more weight. The beauty of this program is that it is adjustable to any fitness level. You can even do it with a friend who may be at a different fitness level than you are and you can both work out at the same time. Have I thought of everything?

There are 4 different full body workouts in the Hot and Healthy Body Program. Exercising 4 days a week is ideal. If you can only get in three days don't worry as long as you keep going. We women need to learn not to be so hard on ourselves. There is no right or wrong just doing and moving forward.

One of the first steps to getting in shape and losing weight is self-love and self-acceptance. I want you from this day forward to promise me that you will only talk to yourself as if you would talk to your friends or children. That means positive, motivating and uplifting words only. Kick any negative thought to the curb.

I always recommend using a calendar that you are going to see everyday and plan out what days you are going to do your exercising on. I recommend putting the calendar on your fridge, bathroom mirror or somewhere where you will see it every day. Cross off the days you exercise with a big X in your favorite color. Once you see these X's adding up you know you are on your way to a Hot and Healthy body. This is a "VISUAL MOTIVATOR" and will help keep you accountable.

I have also included a cardio program for those of you who want to bump it up even more.

At the end of each week I will be sharing with you my "LONDON GEMS". These gems are cutting edge information that you need to know to keep your body functioning in tip top condition for the rest of your life. I call them Gem's because they are topics that I believe you need to know about to live in your Goddess Body and to help you reach your fullest and highest goddess power.

The Workouts:

The workouts start with 3 AB exercises. I love starting with the ABS because it is a great warm up for the whole body. Next, you will move into your circuits. There are three circuits in each workout. Run through the AB circuit before moving on the whole body circuits.

Depending on your ability level run through each circuit one to three times before moving on to the next circuit. Rest when you need it and build up your strength.

Every exercise can be performed at the beginner, intermediate and advanced level. Increase your range of motion, tempo and weight used to increase the difficulty. Challenge yourself and make the mind muscle connection. Don't just do the movements, feel the movements.

Doing the whole routine once should take you about 20 minutes, running through the circuits twice should take you about 40 minutes, running through all the circuits 3 times should take you 60 minutes.

Week 1 Check List:

- Read your Goals everyday

- Journal your food every day

- Journal your thoughts and feelings each day

- Drink up to 64 oz. of quality water

- Perform your circuit workout 3 to 4 times a week

- Mark your workouts with an X on your success calendar

- Weigh yourself and take measurements once a week

- Remove "Franken Foods" from your home

- Add in extra cardio to speed up results

- Nurture Your Inner Goddess by doing something special just for you

- Add a green drink or smoothie to your nutrition plan

- Find one new healthy recipe a week to try

- Enjoy the goddess body you have today and live with passion

What You Need

This is a list of the equipment you are going to need for your Hot and Healthy Workouts. The beauty of the workouts is that you can do them at home or in the gym. Print them out and take them with you or save them to your iPhone or iPad. I have done all these workouts myself and use them with my personal training client so I know they work.

- Water Bottle

- Exercise Mat

- 5 to 15 lb. Weights

- Stability Ball

- Lots of Energy

- Gym Boss Timer (Optional)

I love my Gymboss Timer and use it all the time. They come in all sorts of fun colors.

Week One Exercises

ABS	REPS	SETS
Crunches on stability ball	15	2-3
Push Up Position AB - Knee to Elbow Squeeze	15	2-3
Side Squeeze with Weight	15	2-3

CIRCUIT #1	REPS	SETS	WEIGHT
Alternating Lunge w. Bicep Curl	15 / Leg	2-3	5-15 lbs.
Squat w. Overhead Shoulder Press	15	2-3	5-15 lbs.
Single Leg Dead Lift	15 / Leg	2-3	5-15 lbs.
Jumping Jacks	30 sec.	2-3	Body Weight

CIRCUIT #2	REPS	SETS	WEIGHT
Plié Squat with Upright Shoulder Row	15	2-3	5-15 lbs.
Pendulum Lunges	10 / Leg	2-3	5-15 lbs.
Push Ups on Stability Ball	15	2-3	Body Weight
Squat Hops	30	2-3	Body Weight

CIRCUIT #3	REPS	SETS	WEIGHT
Squat w. Overhead Triceps Extension	15	2-3	5-15 lbs.
Step Ups w. Bicep Hammer Curl	15 / Leg	2-3	5-15 lbs.
Super Woman on the Stability Ball (for the Back)	15	2-3	5-15 lbs.
Flying Lunges	15	2-3	Body Weight

Cardio Program

20-Minute HIIT Cardio (High Intensity Interval Training)

I love High Intensity Training. You get a big bang for your cardio buck here and you know I like to get it in and get it done! You can do this on any cardio equipment or even outside walking, sprinting or running. You will get your heart pumping quickly. Challenge yourself, make it a game and you will have more fun.

Cardio Instructions:

Doing the extra cardio in addition to your circuit workouts will help you to burn fat faster. Keep in mind the workouts I gave you are heart pumping workouts. So if you don't have the time to add in 20 minutes of cardio it's OK. Do cardio on your non circuit days.

Example of HIIT Interval Training

Treadmill or Elliptical

5 minute warm up

Interval Portion

1 minute increase resistance & speed on machine

1 minute reduce resistance & speed = recovery time

1 minute increase resistance & speed on machine

1 minute reduce resistance and speed = recovery time

Repeat the interval sequence 3-4 times

3 minute cool down

Outdoors:

Try 2 minutes of walking, then walk briskly for 30 seconds and then jog/sprint for 30 seconds. Keep alternating. Include a cool down.

For moderate-intensity physical activity, a person's target heart rate should be 50% to 70% of his or her maximum heart rate. This maximum rate is based on the person's age. An estimate of a person's maximum age-related heart rate can be obtained by subtracting the person's age from 220. For example, for a 40-year-old person, the estimated maximum age-related heart rate would be calculated as

220 - 40 years = 180 beats per minute (bpm). Then 50% and 70% levels would be:

50% level: 180 x 0.50 = 90 bpm, and 70% level: 180 x 0.70 = 126 bpm

Exercises Explained: Workout 1

ABS

Crunches on Stability Ball

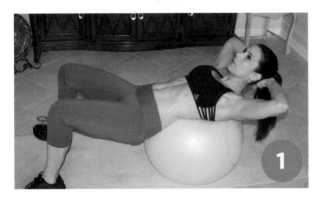
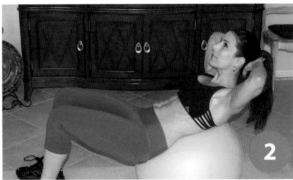

Place lower back on ball. Slowly crunch up. Focus on squeezing the ABS. Lower back down, repeat.

Push Up Position – Knee to AB Elbow Squeeze

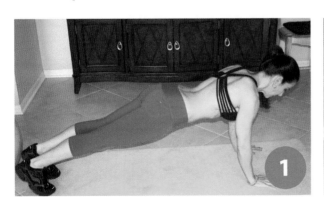
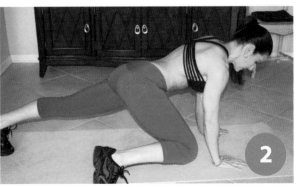

In the push up position bring right knee to outside of right elbow, squeeze. Repeat on opposite side.

Side Squeeze with Weight

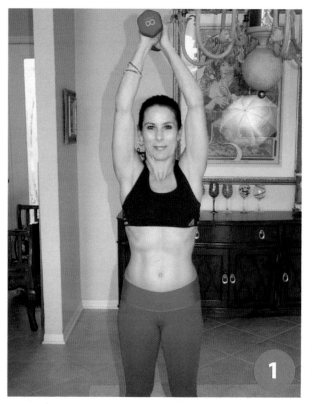 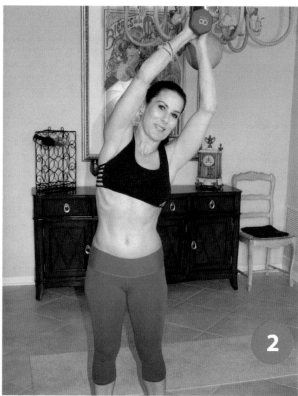

Hold weight overhead, slowly bend to one side, feel the stretch. Return to center, bend to other side.

CIRCUIT 1

Alternating Lunge with Bicep Curl

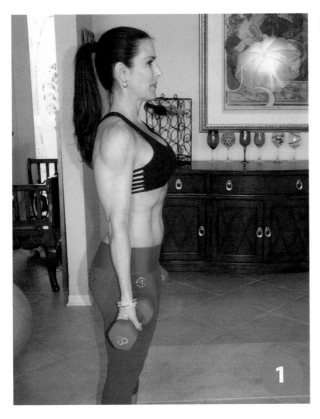 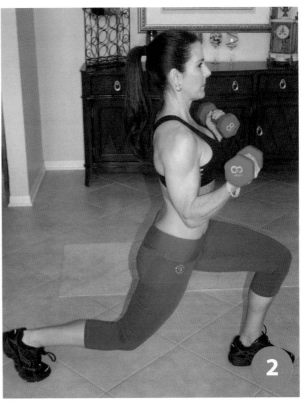

Stand with feet shoulder width apart, palms facing forward. Lunge forward, then do a bicep curl, return to center, repeat on opposite leg. Keep knee in line with toes, do not overextend knee over toes.

Squat With Overhead Shoulder Press

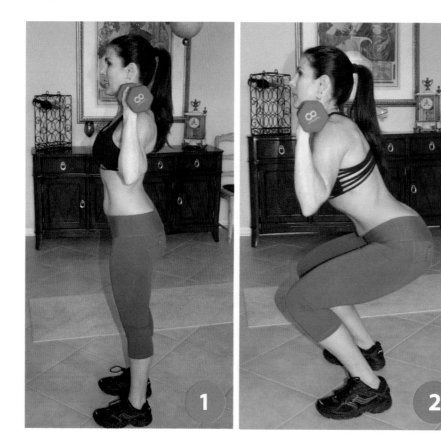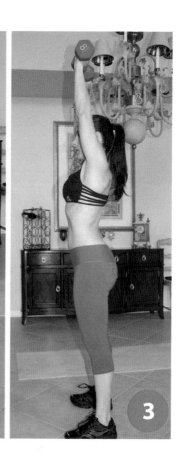

Stand with feet about hip width apart, weights are parallel with shoulders, palms facing forward. Squat down slowly, explosively push up with legs and raise weights overhead at the same time. Repeat

Single Leg Dead Lift

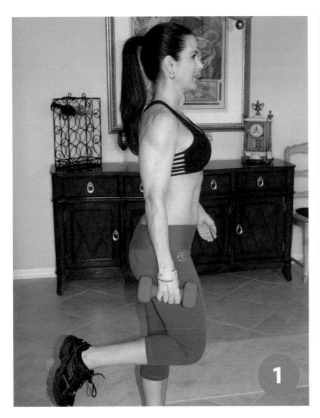

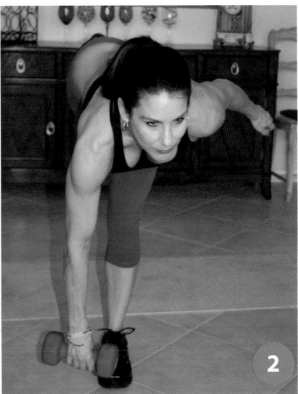

Stand on one leg, hold weight on opposite side, slowly bend forward, feel the stretch in your hamstring. Focus on a spot in front of you, slowly pull yourself back up using your leg not the upper body. Focus.

Jumping Jack

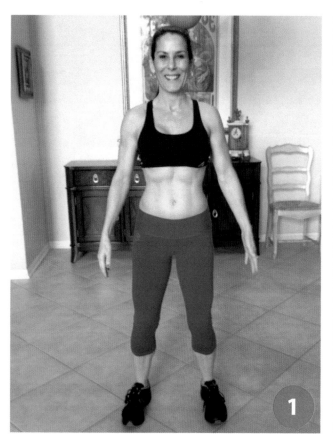
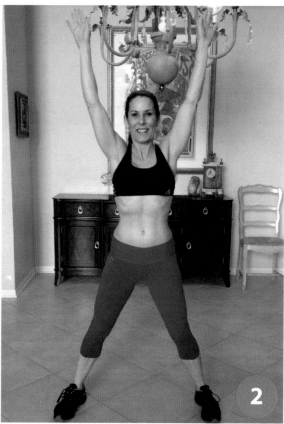

CIRCUIT 2

Plie Squat with Upright Shoulder Row

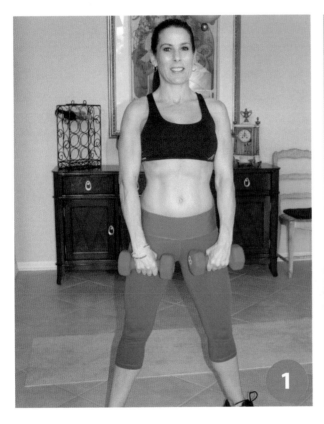
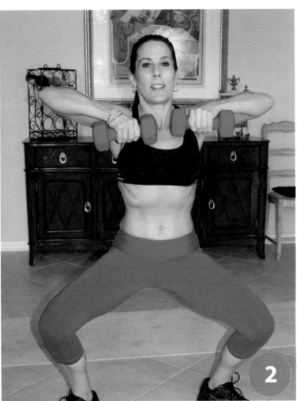

Stand with feet slightly wider than hip width apart. Point toes outward. Weights with palms facing the body. Slowly lower down into a squat, knees pointing outward in line with toes. Feel the inner thigh stretch. Pull weights up to chin, keeping elbows higher than weights. Return weights down. Press legs back up to center. Repeat.

Pendulum Lunge

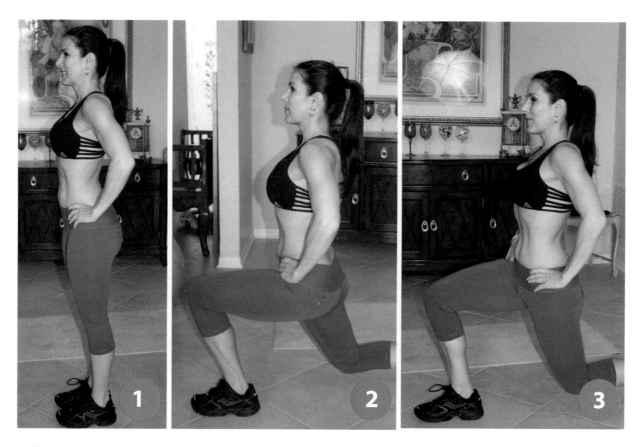

These are great for the thighs. Lunge forward and then sweep leg backward and lunge backward. Return to starting posting.

Push Ups on the Stability ball

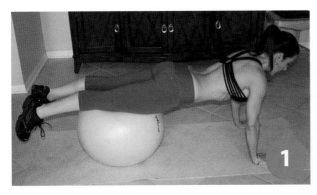 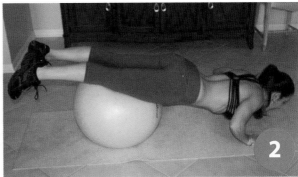

The farther you roll out away from the ball the harder the movement. Great for building upper body strength.

Squat Hops

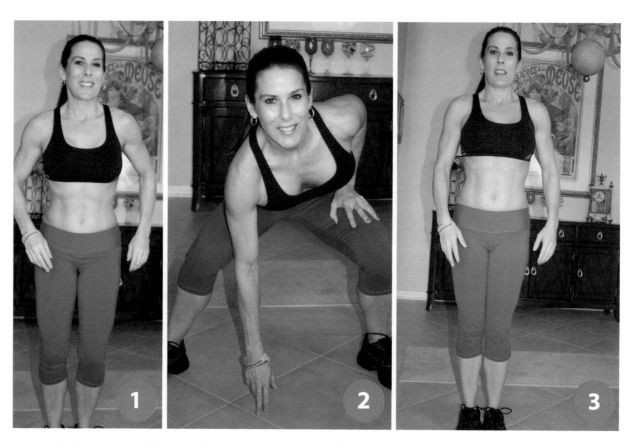

Reach down, touch the floor hop back up, feet together then hop back down touch floor repeat.

CIRCUIT 3

Squat with Overhead Triceps Extension

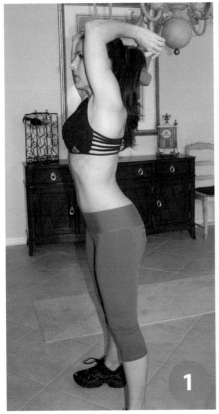 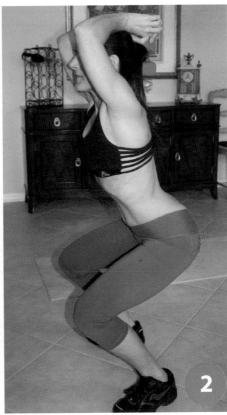 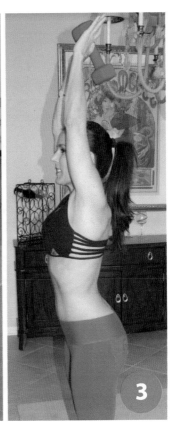

Stand with feet shoulder width apart, hold dumbbell behind head. Squat down and up, then do an overhead triceps extension. Make sure elbows are close to your ears.

Steps Ups with Bicep Hammer Curl

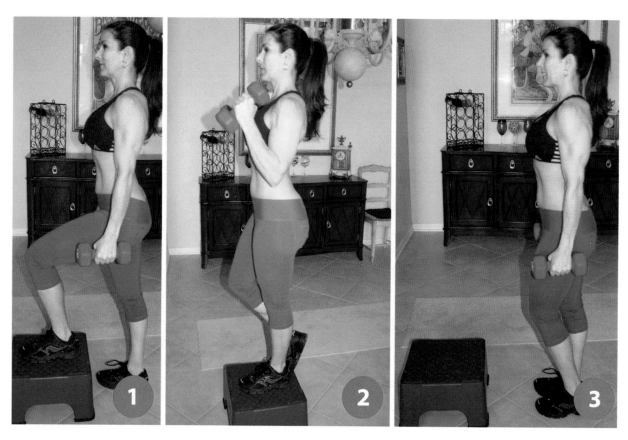

You can use a step in your house or a weight bench. The height of the step will increase the intensity of the exercise. Step up with one leg, perform a bicep hammer curl, tap toe on step and return to floor.

Super Woman on the Stability Ball for the Back

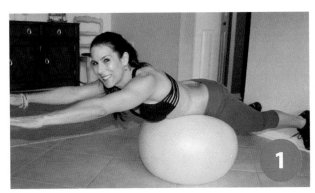 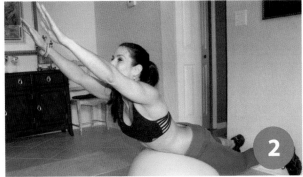

Harder than it looks and it gets your hamstrings too. Place feet against wall for support, abs on the ball. Reach your hands forward and lift the body up. Feel the stretch in your back. Release and repeat.

Flying Lunges

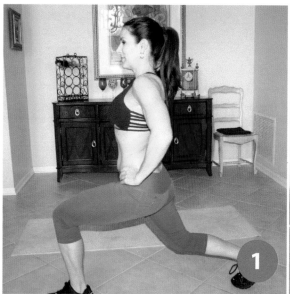
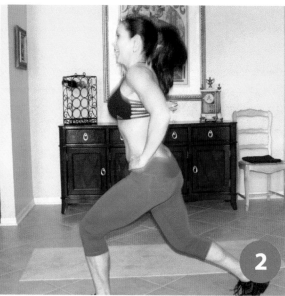
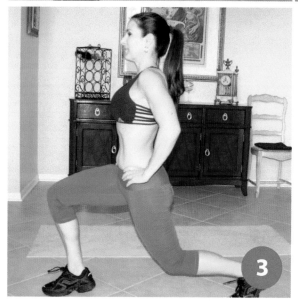

Start in the lunge position with left foot forward. Hop up and flunge by switching legs moving right foot forward and left foot in back. Alternate the flying lunge legs.

London GEM's Week One

In week one we are going to be talking out your Goddess Body and how it functions from the inside out. Weight loss is so much more than just calories in and calories out. Once you truly realize how the body works you will finally have the owner's manual that has been missing. How great is that?

Let Food be Your Medicine and Medicine be Your Food

~ Hippocrates ~

Hello Meet Your Body

In order to be in the best shape of your life it takes more than lifting weights or doing cardio. Once you truly understand your body and how it functions there will be no stopping you.

I am going to go over some very important and cutting edge information. These are the foundations you need to know and understand to reach your goals. For now, I want to open your eyes and your minds to how your body works so you can make significant changes in your life.

I am a "Fitness" professional but my passion has always been nutrition and wellness. People are always asking me what I eat, and what supplements I take. When I tell people I eat real food and my supplements are a green drink and super foods, they look at me with a puzzled look and then repeat the question.

"Did you know the body replaces every cell of your body in 7 years? You can build a whole brand new body"

But we want it quicker than 7 years don't we? I just want you to realize that your body is always replacing new cells. Some live longer than others, but the point is you can build healthy cells from the foods you eat or unhealthy cells from the poor food choices you make, the decision is yours.

Every day your body replaces around 300 BILLION cells, they die off and are

> "Did you know the body replaces every cell of your body in 7 years? You can build a whole brand new body!"

replaced by living cells that are produced at the rate of about 200 million every minute. I will give you one guess what the new cells are made of? Are you ready for this, the food you eat and the thoughts you think!

Cells only need three simple things to survive and thrive

Food- Water - Air

Knowing this information, why in the world would you want to build unhealthy cells? Unhealthy cells lead to all sorts of diseases and ailments. Imagine you are building a brand new house, wouldn't you want to pick the finest quality

> *"...it is not normal to wake up in the morning tired and groggy and needing a "fix" of caffeine to get your day moving..."*

materials, the best of everything?

So lets do this for your body too. You are the builder, the architect of your body. Guess what? You also have a major influence on the ones you love, your friends and family.

So lets get started to learn about some key information that is going to change the way you think about DIET forever.

Live a Vibrant and Healthy Life

I am going to briefly go over some very important information that everyone needs to know in order to live a healthy, vibrant life full of energy and vitality.

Do you find yourself doing things like this? You decide that you are going to lose weight. You buy healthy food, start exercising. You can start to see and feel the benefits of your new eating and exercise plan. You are excited and feeling proud of yourself and then a few weeks later your old habits start creeping back in.

You decide to skip a workout, go out to dinner with friends and instead of eating a delicious and healthy meal you go overboard and eat everything in sight and wake up the next day with a food hangover? You know what I am talking about. Your eyes are swollen, your body feels stiff and you just feel awful. That is what I call a food hangover.

Then you think what's the use, I am just a "big girl". I was meant to be this way. Do you beat yourself up for not being strict enough to stay on your "diet".

Do you wonder why you can be doing so well and feeling great and then all of a sudden, WHAM! You fall off the wagon and beat yourself up about it?

One of the reasons is because diets don't work. They are a temporary solution to an underlying issue. I am going to help you finally understand what is keeping you from being successful and having everything you truly desire.

Did you know it is not normal to wake up in the morning tired and groggy and needing a "fix" of caffeine to get your day moving? It is your birthright to feel healthy, happy and full of energy every morning when you wake up.

I am going to finally help you understand the real reason as to what is holding you back from reaching not only your weight loss goals but how to improve the quality of your life and that of the ones you love.

I am going to teach you how to take charge of your health once and for all and start living the life you were meant to live.

Do you want to learn the secret to natural permanent weight loss with the least amount of effort possible? Do you want to learn how to increase your energy by 50% without having to rely on caffeine or sugar anymore?

I want you to stand up and shout YES I AM READY! Now if you are in a room full of people this may not be the best thing to do for obvious reasons.

I want you to stand up anyway and just scream it silently, in your head YES, I AM READY! Did you get a big smile across your face? I know you did, because taking charge feels good and you deserve it.

Hello, Meet Your Hormones

Hi, I would like to introduce you to your best friend or your worst enemy.

Ok, the "H" word. This is a BIG ONE and one of the most important chapters of this book. This, ladies, is going to rock your world.

Deep inside you know this information. Why? Because you are a woman, and hormones truly rule our world from the time we get up in the morning until the time we go to bed. You can't ever really fully explain the highs and lows we go through to a man, but after you read this you are going to scream YES!! It all makes sense now.

The majority of fitness programs out there today are designed for "men" and then adjusted for a women to follow them too. They are designed and marketed by men who forget one very important fact. We are women and our bodies function totally different.

Not only are we built differently, we store fat differently, burn calories differently and have a totally different set of hormones than a man does. Now please understand I "love" men and I am in no way putting them down. I am just pointing out an overlooked issue when it comes to designing fitness programs for women.

Here is a great example of what I am talking about. When I first started to compete in figure competitions I trained with a trainer. The very first trainer I ever used was a woman. Let's call her Allison. Allison was a fitness competitor at the time and I remember seeing her in a copy of the fitness magazine, Oxygen.

Now this was someone I really wanted to learn from. She had a beautifully sculpted body, she was always full of energy and I loved learning from her. Her training was great. Do you know why? Because she trained me like a woman.

She could sense there were weeks when I had more energy and was on top of the world and would take advantage of this and really challenge me in my workout sessions.

Then there were weeks when I just did not have that much energy, I would be tired and dragging and again she adjusted the workout.

The results of training with her were amazing. My body was toned and fit but in a sexy way. I still had womanly curves and did not lose my femininity. Many of the other competitors on stage had a more square look to them and had lost their womanly shape.

I believe this was because they were women, training like men. I went on to win three first place titles that year, a major accomplishment never having competed before.

When I started to compete a few years later, my new trainer was a young, smart and very knowledgeable man. But this time something was different. My body looked different. I had a lot of muscle but was looking more square and had lost my sexy curves.

The training was way too intense and I did not have the same figure when I stepped on stage that I once had. The whole point of this story is just to show you that a man and a woman's body are very different when it comes to diet and exercise and it all comes down to hormones.

Can women have success with men trainers? Of course they can and they do.

But I know you will be more successful, and achieve faster and greater results when you understand how to work with and not against your hormones.

There Is A Party And I Am Not Invited?

Does this sound familiar to you? You decided to start a nutrition and exercise plan. You are doing a great job, exercising, eating well, and you think to yourself, this is it, this is the time I am going to be successful. I am going to stick to my diet and exercise plan and finally have the figure I have wanted for a long time.

You are planning your meals, starting to feel better and then you think, it's not happening fast enough or you find yourself losing your drive and falling off the wagon. You think, what happened? I was doing so well and then all of a sudden BAM, it happened again, those negative thoughts come in your head. I can't do this, I have no self control, no willpower.

You find yourself running into the drugstore for a candy bar or two or is it the drive through for french fries or maybe a bag of potato chips at the grocery store. You eat them and then feel so upset with yourself.

You want to cry, "why can't I just control my eating" ?

Maybe you do fine for a while and then all of a sudden you just feel down, you just want to curl up in a blanket, and shut the world out.

You beat yourself up and then give up, thinking, "What's the use, I can't do it, just forget the whole thing. I am just supposed to be like this. What is the use?"

What if I told you it is not your fault? Would that make you feel better? It happens to so many women across the world. They have the best intentions and then something seems to stop their progress. Well, it is not a secret anymore. It is your HORMONES.

Your hormones are out of control, having a wild party in your body every month and they forgot to invite you!

Now that you know about the party, it's time for you to take charge and be the party planner of your own body.

Are You Going To Eat That Cookie or Should I?

Cravings and out of control hunger are a big sign that your hormones are at their highest concentration during your monthly cycle. All of a sudden you find yourself switching from carrots and grilled chicken, which you were enjoying to craving chocolate, salty chips or ice cream.

This is because your body is low in serotonin at this time of the month and it is sending out signals to get more. The quickest way for us to get this "feel good" hormone is to eat carbs. This is why we get those uncontrollable cravings or just seem twice as hungry than we normally are. It is not that you don't have strong enough will power; it is your body sending signals out to eat more.

The best way to be in control of these cravings, are to first realize the reason why it is happening.

"Now that you know it's not because you are losing your willpower but it is a hormone shift in your body you can deal with it in a different way."

Which Carb Do You Crave?

Sweet, salty, savory, smooth & creamy, crunchy, cake or cookies or just anything that has chocolate in it? Think about what you crave and write down a healthy alternative here so you will be prepared.

I crave _____

A healthy alternative I will use is_____

Now we are going to have a plan of attack and by having healthy alternative carbs on hand to satisfy or "crowd out" these cravings and knowing it is OK to give into them is going to help a lot. Planning a preparation is key to being successful in managing those cravings when they hit.

For me it is chocolate. I love anything with chocolate. My healthy alternative at first was a chocolate chip Vita Muffin or a gluten free Chocolate Muffin. I found this satisfies my chocolate craving and was quick and easy. I was satisfied after eating it and felt better knowing I had a healthy choice instead.

Once the craving is satisfied I am fine and can go on normally. Before I would try to deny myself chocolate, but what would happen instead would be that chocolate was all I could think about and I would have to eat it and then overindulge in it.

At a very low point in my life I remember making up excuses to go to the grocery store, like we are out of eggs, just so I could go buy chocolate and eat it in my car so no one would know. Sound familiar? Deprivation and hormones do not work. The hormones will win just about every time.

So I urge you to go and start to find a healthy replacement for when those crazy cravings hit. Now I make my own homemade chocolate healthy muffins and have them in the freezer for when the chocolate monster arrives.

Exercise 101
Week 2

Here we are at week two already! How did week one go for you? Are you reading your Why and your goals every day? Remember it's super important to read them. How many days of the week did you exercise? Use your calendar to cross off those days you do your circuit workouts and any additional exercising. When you see those X's adding up you know you are on your way to your Hot and Healthy Body.

Let's talk about your nutrition program. What changes did you make this week? Were you consistent in writing down and journaling the foods you ate? This is key to being successful in the first 30 days. Are you drinking enough water? Remember we need to keep that Goddess Body hydrated for it to function efficiently. Plus it makes your skin glow, helps to reduce fine lines, cuts down on cravings and helps to detoxify the body. Go get a glass of water now.

Are you sleeping better this past week? Sleeping beauty was pretty darn smart. Sleep is such an overlooked KEY to losing weight. There is a lot of research going on about your appetite, hormones and how sleep plays a large role in weight loss. Turn off the TV or computer before bed, relax and read a book or have a conversation with someone you love. Learn how to shut down your body at night. Lavender essential oil is great to relax and calm the body for rest. You can put a drop on your hands and breath it in, diffuse it in the air and even add a drop to your pillow for a restful nights sleep.

Did you enjoy reading week one's London Fit Gems? Are you realizing that your hormones play a major role in how you feel, weight loss and your cravings? That you really do have control and once you make friends with your hormones weight loss will be easier. My job is to educate you on how your body works. Once I do this you will have all the tools you need for success and a rocking Hot and Healthy Body.

I am so excited for you to start week two. You have a brand new full body circuit workout this week. Just when your body was getting used to weeks ones workout we are going to change it up. Keep that body guessing and use different movements and different muscle combinations to get a Hot and Healthy Body.

Guess what? You have new London Gems to read about this week. Think of it as your homework only this is for pure enjoyment and there are no tests! This week we are going to learn about your body's "second brain". Bet you did not know you had two brains! Digestion, enzymes and their importance in weight loss. How adding green smoothies to your diet will make your skin radiant, and superfoods to add to take your Hot and Healthy nutrition to the next level.

Run through your checklist every day to stay on track and have a great week!

Week 2 Check List:

- Read your Goals everyday

- Journal your food every day

- Journal your thoughts and feelings each day

- Drink up to 64 oz. of quality water

- Perform your circuit workout 3 to 4 times a week

- Mark your workouts with an X on your success calendar

- Weigh yourself and take measurements once a week

- Remove "Franken Foods" from your home

- Add in extra cardio to speed up results

- Nurture Your Inner Goddess by doing something special just for you

- Add a green drink or smoothie to your nutrition plan

- Find one new healthy recipe a week to try

- Enjoy the goddess body you have today and live with passion

The Workouts:

The workouts start with 3 AB exercises. I love starting with the ABS because it is a great warm up for the whole body. Next you will move into your circuits. There are three circuits in each workout. Run through the AB circuit before moving on the whole body circuits.

Depending on your ability level run through each circuit one to three times before moving on to the next circuit. Rest when you need it and build up your strength.

Every exercise can be performed at the beginner, intermediate and advanced level. Increase your range of motion, tempo and weight used to increase the difficulty. Challenge yourself and make the mind muscle connection. Don't just do the movements, feel the movements.

Doing the whole routine once should take you about 20 minutes. Running through the circuits twice should take you about 40 minutes. Running through all the circuits 3 times should take you 60 minutes.

What You Need

This is a list of the equipment you are going to need for your Hot and Healthy Workouts. The beauty of the workouts is that you can do them at home or in the gym. Print them out and take them with you or save them to your iPhone or iPad. I have done all these workouts myself and use them with my personal training clients, so I know they work.

- Water Bottle

- Exercise Mat

- 5 to 15 lb. Weights

- Stability Ball

- Lots of Energy

- Gym Boss Timer (Optional)

I love my Gymboss Timer and use it all the time. They come in all sorts of fun colors.

Week Two
Exercises

ABS	REPS	SETS
Wall Stability Ball AB Crunches	15	2-3
Stability Ball AB Exchange	15	2-3
Oblique AB Twist on Stability Ball	15	2-3

CIRCUIT #1	REPS	SETS	WEIGHT
Booty Blast to The Sky	20 / Leg	2-3	Ankle weights *optional
Squat with a Side Kick & Over Head Shoulder Press	20	2-3	5-15 lbs.
Stability Ball Booty Hip Lift & Pulses	20 Lifts 20 Pulses	2-3	Body Weight
Toe Taps	30 sec.	2-3	

CIRCUIT #2	REPS	SETS	WEIGHT
Squat, Hammer Curl & Over Head Shoulder Press	15	2-3	5-15 lbs.
Stationary Lunge with Over Head Shoulder Hold	10 / Leg	2-3	5-15 lbs.
Dead Lift with Front Raise & Over Head Raise	15	2-3	5-15 lbs.

CIRCUIT #3	REPS	SETS	WEIGHT
Inner Thigh Plié Squats with Side Shoulder Raise	15	2-3	5-15 lbs.
Criss Cross Squats	15 / Leg	2-3	5-15 lbs.
Stability Ball Booty Hip Lift & Lying Triceps Extensions	15	2-3	5-15 lbs.

Cardio Program

20-Minute HIIT Cardio (High Intensity Interval Training)

I love High Intensity Training. You get a big bang for your cardio buck here and you know I like to get it in and get it done! You can do this on any cardio equipment or even outside walking, sprinting or running. You will get your heart pumping quickly. Challenge yourself, make it a game and you will have more fun.

Cardio Instructions:

Doing the extra cardio in addition to your circuit workouts will help you to burn fat faster. Keep in mind the workouts I gave you are heart pumping workouts. So if you don't have the time to add in 20 minutes of cardio it's OK. Do cardio on your non-circuit days.

Example of HIIT Interval Training

Treadmill or Elliptical

5 minute warm up

Interval Portion

1 minute increase resistance & speed on machine

1 minute reduce resistance & speed = recovery time

1 minute increase resistance & speed on machine

1 minute reduce resistance and speed = recovery time

Repeat the interval sequence 3-4 times

3 minute cool down

Outdoors:

Try 2 minutes of walking, then walk briskly for 30 seconds and then jog/sprint for 30 seconds. Keep alternating. Include a cool down.

For moderate-intensity physical activity, a person's target heart rate should be 50% to 70% of his or her maximum heart rate. This maximum rate is based on the person's age. An estimate of a person's maximum age-related heart rate can be obtained by subtracting the person's age from 220. For example, for a 40-year-old person, the estimated maximum age-related heart rate would be calculated as

220 - 40 years = 180 beats per minute (bpm). Then 50% and 70% levels would be:

50% level: 180 x 0.50 = 90 bpm, and 70% level: 180 x 0.70 = 126 bpm

Exercises Explained: Workout 2

ABS

Wall Stability Ball AB Crunches

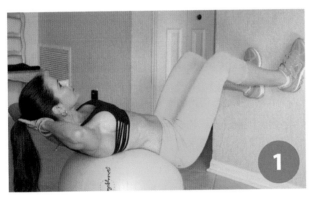 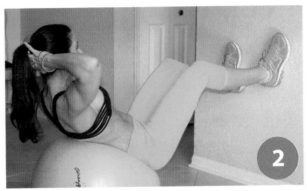

A different twist on the AB crunch. Place feet on the wall and crunch up slowly. Focus on the AB Muscles working.

Stability Ball AB Exchange

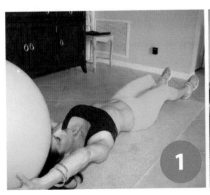 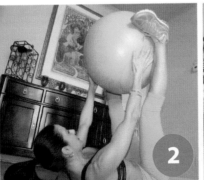 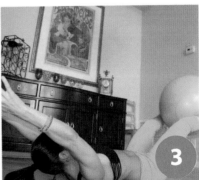

Lie on your back, arms and legs outstretched. With stability ball in hands reach ball up to center to meet legs. Crunch and exchange stability ball to feet. Lower arms and legs trying not to touch the ground and keep tension on your abs. Repeat exchange.

Oblique Ab Twist on Stability Ball

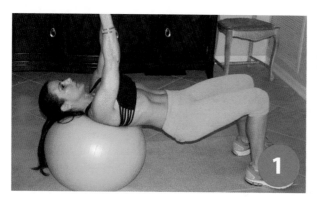 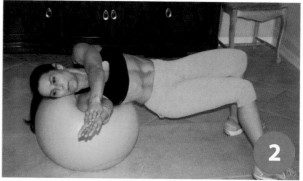

Center, Twist Right, Center, Twist Left. Slow and Controlled feel the squeeze in the Obliques. Add weight to challenge yourself.

CIRCUIT 1

Booty Blast to the Sky

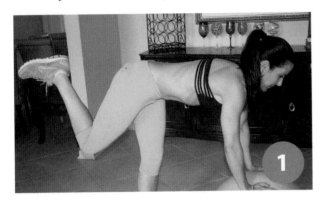 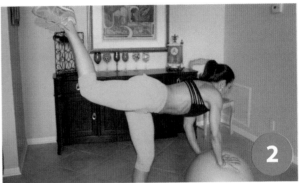

The heel is going up to the ceiling. Picture, balancing a book on your foot.

Squat with Side Kick & Over Head Shoulder Press

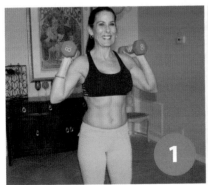 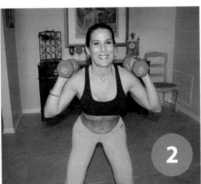 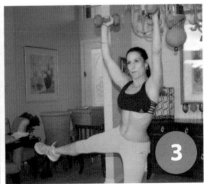

Hold weights above shoulders. Feet hip width apart. Squat down then explode up pushing the weights over your head and kicking leg out to the side alternating legs.

Stability Ball Booty Hip Lifts & Pulses

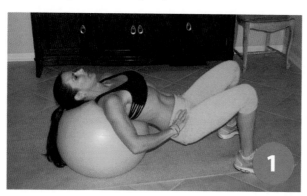 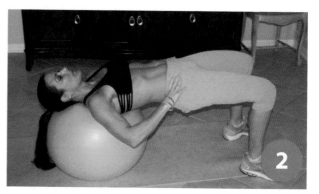

Rest head and upper shoulders on stability ball. Drop hips close to the floor. Lift hips up to the ceiling and squeeze the booty. Repeat for 20. Then keeping hips up to ceiling do 20 quick booty squeezes.

Toe Taps – Tap Toes Back & Forth

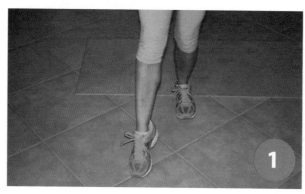 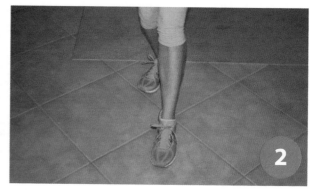

Quickly tap your feet front and back alternating at a fast pace. This is a 30 second exercise to get your heart rate pumping.

CIRCUIT 2

Squat, Hammer Curl & Overhead Shoulder Press

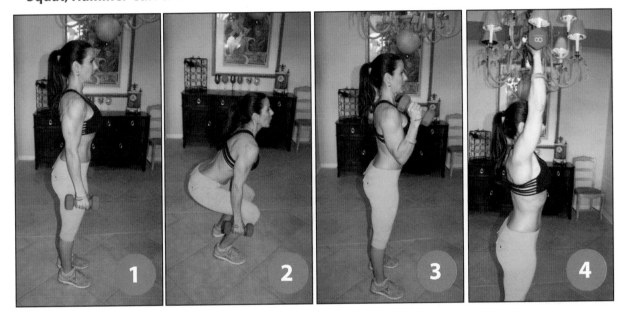

Stationary Lunge with Overhead Shoulder Hold

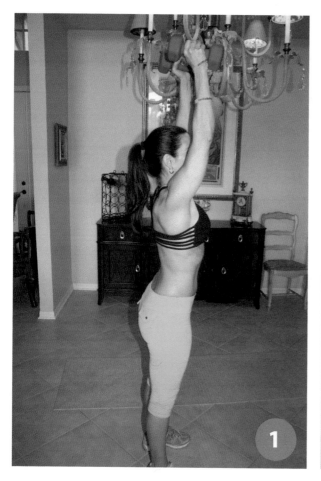 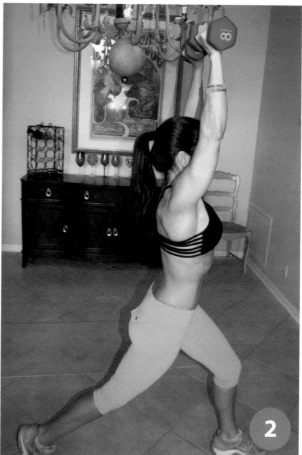

Hold Arms Above Shoulder for the Whole Exercise, Lunge forward, then dip down and up for 10 then switch legs.

Dead Lift with Shoulder Front Raise & Overhead Lift

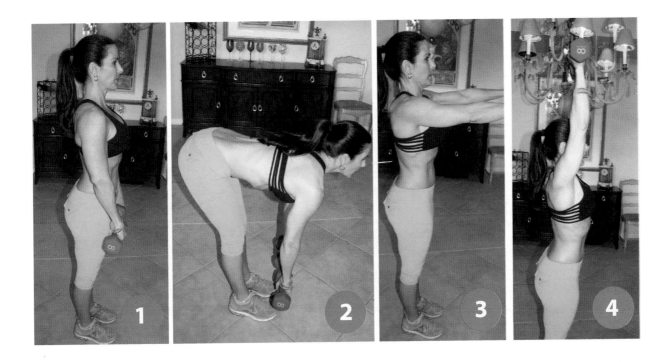

Stand with feel shoulder width apart, bend down, feel the stretch in your hamstrings. Focus pulling up using your glutes (not the upper body). When standing, do a front shoulder raise lifting weights up and then over your head and return back down. Repeat

CIRCUIT 3

Inner Thigh Plie Squats with Side Shoulder Raise

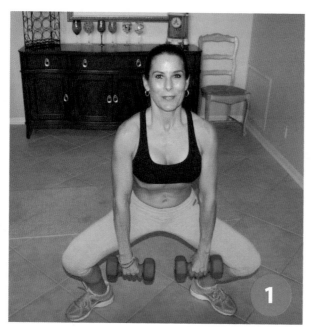 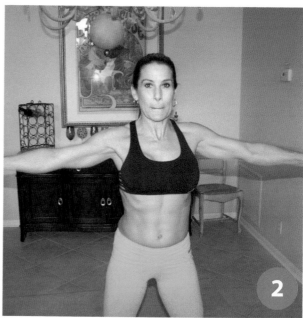

Point toes outward, squat down making sure knees are going out over toes, feel the inner thigh stretch. Push up into a shoulder side raise.

Criss Cross Squats

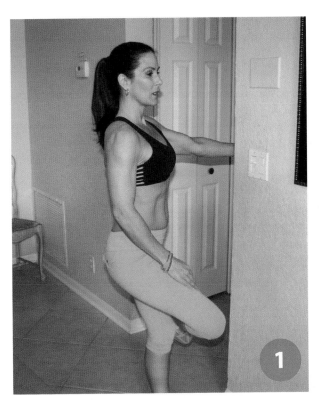
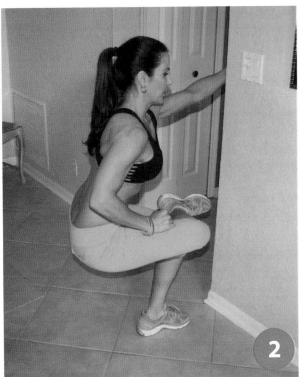

Hold on to something sturdy, cross leg over thigh, slowly lower yourself down. Feel the stretch in the hip area, push up through heel. Make the booty work.

Stability Ball Booty Hip Lifts & Lying Triceps Extensions

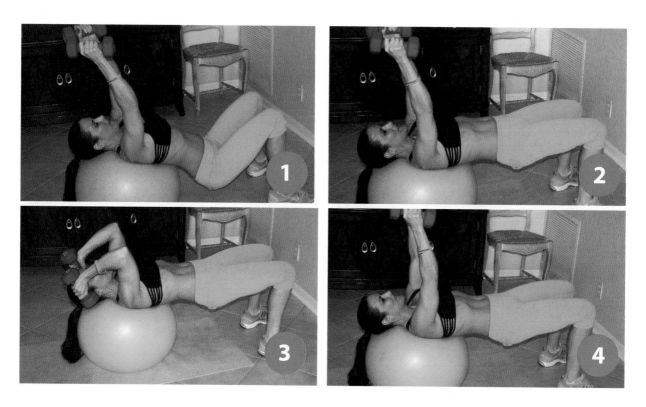

Head & neck on the ball. Arms extended up over head. Drop booty to floor, then squeeze up to ceiling. Then lower weights to side of head, extend back up repeat. Booty squeeze, triceps extension.

Low Frog Hops

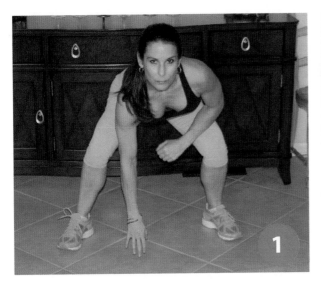 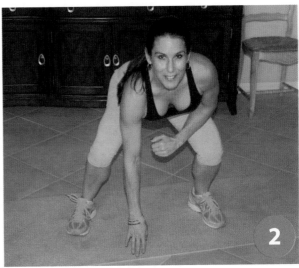

Bend down in a squat position. Jump forward keeping as low as you can and then jump backwards keep it going for 30 seconds.

London GEM's Week Two

Welcome to week two. You are doing a great job. This week we are going to learn about digestion and your second brain. We will learn here digestion really starts. It is not where you think! The amazing benefits of adding green smoothies and essential oils to your nutrition plan to make your skin glow and your body hot and healthy from the inside out.

Are you ready to learn even more about your Goddess Body? Did you rush over to this section to see what I have in store for you in week two? Remember weight loss is not just about exercising and eating less. It is about understanding how your body works and why.

This week we are going to be focusing on our digestion and why it is KEY in weight loss. We are going to learn about enzymes, why we need them and how they will help you lose weight. I am going to introduce you to your second brain. Bet you did not even know you had two brains. Don't worry it will all make sense soon.

Probiotics and the foods that they come from naturally. The amazing benefits of fermented foods. Why goddess green smoothies are a girls best friend. The superfoods I recommend for gorgeous skin and hair.

It's a lot of great information so get comfy and read on.

Enzymes & Digestion

Statistics show that our country has a terrible problem with vitamin and enzyme deficiency. Think about how many fruits and vegetables you really eat in a day? I bet your diet is mainly made up of cooked foods. Am I right?

Living foods are foods that are not cooked such as, apples, oranges, carrots, lettuce. You get the picture. These living foods are bursting with nutrition and living enzymes. Prolonged cooking, processing and pasteurization destroy the enzymes necessary to break down foods properly.

> *"Statistics show that our country has a terrible problem with vitamin and enzyme deficiency."*

A quick overview of the three digestive enzymes:

Protease to digest protein – Digestion of proteins is mainly done in the stomach. Proteins are long, twisted chains that need to be broken down before they can be used by the body.

Amylases to digest carbohydrates/starch – This enzyme is found in our saliva and it is the first step in the digestion of carbohydrates.

Lipase to digest fats – This enzyme is used to break down fat mainly in the small intestines.

> "We are born with a certain amount of enzyme and the more cooked foods we eat the more the body has to call on its reserves of enzymes."

These three enzymes help the body to break down food so it can be absorbed in the small intestine. Live enzymes are the catalyst for every human function. Think of them as little energy cheerleaders. You want as many cheerleaders jumping up and down and giving you as much energy as you can get. The more cooked food we eat, the more we deplete our body of these precious "cheerleader" enzymes.

We are born with a certain amount of enzyme and the more cooked foods we eat the more the body has to call on its reserves of enzymes. Think about how you feel after you eat a large dinner. Don't you feel tired? This is because if your meal was mainly made of cooked foods, your body is working hard to digest what you just ate. It takes the body more energy to digest food than any other bodily function. It is calling on your precious enzyme reserves.

The good news is that we can help the body by infusing it with living enzymes, which are found in fruits and vegetables. The more living foods we eat equals more enzymes, which equal more energy.

The beauty of fruits and vegetables is that they naturally come with all the enzymes needed for digestion. Look at a beautiful red apple. It is bursting with energy and living enzymes ready to give nutrients to our body.

We directly take in the energy from the food we eat. Now what if we took that very same apple, cooked it in the oven for 30 minutes to make a baked apple? We have killed off all the live enzymes by cooking it and have also taken away most of the nutritional value of the apple.

The point I am trying to make is the more cooked food we eat the less life we have in our own bodies. You all know the saying you are what you eat.

Build your new 300 billion cells with as much living food as possible everyday,. It will love you back. Easy ways to do this are by adding juices, green smoothies, salads, nuts and seeds and raw fruits and veggies to your daily diet.

I explained to you before that there are three different enzymes to break down food, amylase, protease and lipase. Lets look at lipase for example. If you eat an avocado it comes with the lipase enzyme already in it helping the body to break down the fat. But say you use olive oil and cook it at a high temperature, you are killing the lipase enzymes and the body has to draw on its enzyme reserves, taking more energy away from you and putting it toward digestion.

Enzyme Summary

You are born with a certain amount of enzymes for life. Eating cooked food draws on those enzyme reserves. The more living foods, like fruits and vegetables in your diet the healthier you will become.

Living Foods = More Living Enzymes = More Energy + Better Quality of Life

Probiotics & Gut Health

A healthy gut is essential to a healthy body. Did you know your body had two "Brains"? One that we all know about in our head and the other in our GUT. Yes, our gut.

You GUT is an amazing, intelligent part of your body. It is also known as your second brain. If you want the scientific version, it's called the Enteric Nervous

System, or the ENS.

Think about the phrases: go with your GUT, or trust your GUT instincts. Your gut has over 1 million neurons; it records experiences and responds to emotions. The gut's brain is also known to play a major role in human happiness and misery.

What I am trying to tell you is your GUT already knows what foods are good for you and what you should be eating, which means so do you! You just need to tune into it and listen.

Probiotics are a must in digestive health. Taking antibiotics, not digesting food properly, and stress all lead to a gut that is off balance. Antibiotics kill not only the bad bacteria but all the good bacteria too.

When we are in an optimal state of health we should have about 80 to 85 percent friendly bacteria in our digestive tract. The years of taking medication, eating processed and a diet of mainly cooked food all lead to an overbalance of unfriendly bacteria in our system. When this happens we get all sorts of symptoms, gas bloating, indigestion, skin eruptions, lack of energy, digestive issues and many other symptoms.

I highly recommend adding in probiotics to your diet everyday. In the form of supplements and fermented foods.

Fermented foods are full of living enzymes and probiotics that have a beneficial effect on our overall health. I enjoy a fermented drink called Kevita, made from fermented coconut, which you can find in the health food stores and some grocery stores now carry it. Some other fermented food to try and experiment with are kimchi, kombucha, miso and raw apple cider vinegar. Have fun and your digestion will thank you.

Green Goddess Smoothies

OK, by now you have figured out that I am pretty "green & natural". One way to improve your health is to add more greens into your diet. Remember greens are full of living enzymes, and living enzymes equal better digestion and better digestion equal more energy. I think you are getting it now.

One easy way to add more fruit and veggies into your diet is to add the Green Goddess smoothie. I like to call it "Goddess" because we should all be treating ourselves like we are goddesses (or gods, if you're a guy). We deserve it and need to show ourselves more self love.

You can have a "Goddess Smoothie" for any meal. It could be breakfast; this is a great way to start the day. It is easy on digestions because it is mainly predigested and won't take a lot of energy from your body.

Breakfast really means, "break the fast". Your body had been fasting and repairing itself all night. Working on getting rid of toxins, replacing old cells and working hard to repair the damage that has been caused by daily normal living. A Goddess Green Smoothie is a great way to break the fast and get some instant energy and nutrition.

Here is a simple recipe. I have so many more delicious recipes to share with you in my holistic coaching program. I know these smoothies are going to be a go to staple for you once you try them.

Hot & Healthy Recipes

Breakfast: Avocado & Banana Surprise Smoothie

1 medium avocado peeled
1 orange peeled
1/2 frozen banana
1 cup unsweetened almond milk
1 scoop vanilla protein powder
1 to 1 ½ cup water
Cinnamon to taste or cinnamon essential oil
Add a few drops of liquid stevia if you like it sweeter

Lunch: Chicken, hummus and veggie wrap

6 inch whole grain or brown rice wrap
(I like to warm it up just a touch so it is pliable)
½ cut up chicken breast (or go veggie and leave out the chicken)
2 tbsp. hummus
Romaine or mixed baby lettuce
Chopped tomatoes and cucumbers
Grated carrots and zucchini
¼ cup hummus

Dinner: Artichoke Salmon

Wild Caught Salmon
Can also use chicken, tofu or eggplant to change it up
1 jar quartered artichoke hearts in water drained
1 can diced tomatoes with spices (*look for BPA free cans)
Organic spinach
Fresh pressed garlic
Olive oil

DIRECTIONS:

Heat oven to 350 degrees. Place salmon in pan, pour artichokes over salmon, then add the diced tomatoes. Place in oven and cook for about 30 minutes. It will make the most delicious, moist and tasty salmon.

I love to take organic spinach sautee it with a little olive oil and fresh pressed garlic and place the salmon on top. Dinner is done and it makes a great lunch for the next day too!

Snack: Organic corn tortilla chips with natural salsa or hummus

Organic Apple with a handful of your favorite nuts
1 free range hardboiled egg and an orange
Natural low sugar protein bar. I like the Raw Crunch Bar

Love Me Lime Smoothie

1 cucumber peeled
½ avocado
½ cup water or coconut water
2 handfuls spinach
2 limes peeled
Dash of cinnamon
Stevia if desired

Great SUPERFOODS to add in are:

Goji Berries & All Berries
Bee Pollen
Ground Flax Seeds
Chia Seeds
Ashwagandah Root Powder
Maca Powder
Sprouts
Raw Cacao
Cinnamon
Turmeric
Spirulina
Mushrooms
Green Tea
Kale, Spinach, Greens
Green Powder
Nuts & Seeds
Raw Wheat Germ
Nut Butters

Turn up the nutrition by adding in a scoop of a "Green Powder" for additional health benefits. I love to put a peeled organic cucumber in mine every day.

Add all ingredients to blender. Blend and enjoy! Think how many living enzymes you are giving your precious "Goddess" body. You can almost feel the electricity of all the nutrition flowing through your body as you drink it.

Exercise 101
Week 3

We are halfway there!! The time is going by so fast and I know you are doing a great job! You are learning so much about how your beautiful body works and how to take care of it for a lifetime. Are you finally ready to kick dieting to the curb? Be done with it forever? Let's banish it to another galaxy. It's time to feed the body high quality nutrition, superfoods and love it from the inside out. Doesn't that sound like a much better plan? I know it does.

In weeks one and two you have been building some great new habits that will last a lifetime. You are learning to journal your foods, write down your why and read your goals every day. You are speaking to yourself with positive words and thinking uplifting thoughts. Loving the skin you are in today and of course working that beautiful body with the Hot and Healthy circuit workouts.

You are starting to have more energy, you are sleeping better and you no longer have food hangovers in the morning, inflammation is going away. Most important you are listening to your body and tuning in to what it really needs. The body knows; you just have to listen.

You know I have a brand new circuit workout for you! Are you ready to step it up this week? Turn up the fat burning by adding some more resistance to the workouts by increasing your weights. Doing this is really going to challenge your muscles to work harder. Turn up the fat burning even more by adding in some extra cardio. It could be a spin class, maybe Zumba or jump on the treadmill and push the incline button up to a level you have never done before. This is where I want you to dig deep and find that extra energy and motivation.

Week three is where most people will give up. DON'T be one of them. Remember the 10 Steps to Prepare for Success in the beginning of the book? One of them was FINISH WHAT YOU START. Don't give into excuses, not this time. See it through and be committed to yourself and your health. I am here for you! Think of me as your personal trainer and cheerleader all in one. I want you to succeed, I know you can succeed. Just keep going; that is all I am asking.

This week's London Gems are full of great information. You are going to meet your "stress hormone". Her name is Cortisol. Learn about alkalizing the body and why it is so important to weight loss. And my secret weapon for baby soft skin.

Have a great week three and I can't wait to share with you what I have in store for week 4.

Week 3 Check List:

- Read your Goals everyday

- Journal your food every day

- Journal your thoughts and feelings each day

- Drink up to 64 oz. of quality water

- Perform your circuit workout 3 to 4 times a week

- Mark your workouts with an X on your success calendar

- Weigh yourself and take measurements once a week

- Remove "Franken Foods" from your home

- Add in extra cardio to speed up results

- Nurture Your Inner Goddess by doing something special just for you

- Add a green drink or smoothie to your nutrition plan

- Find one new healthy recipe a week to try

- Enjoy the goddess body you have today and live with passion

The Workouts:

The workouts start with 3 AB exercises. I love starting with the ABS because it is a great warm up for the whole body. Next you will move into your circuits. There are three circuits in each workout. Run through the AB circuit before moving on to the whole body circuits.

Depending on your ability level run through each circuit one to three times before moving on to the next circuit. Rest when you need it and build up your strength.

Every exercise can be performed at the beginner, intermediate and advanced level. Increase your range of motion, tempo and weight used to increase the difficulty. Challenge yourself and make the mind muscle connection. Don't just do the movements. Feel the movements.

Doing the whole routine once should take you about 20 minutes, running through the circuits twice should take you about 40 minutes, running through all the circuits 3 times should take you 60 minutes.

What You Need

This is a list of the equipment you are going to need for your Hot and Healthy Workouts. The beauty of the workouts is that you can do them at home or in the gym. Print them out and take them with you or save them to your iPhone or iPad. I have done all these workouts myself and use them with my personal training clients, so I know they work.

- Water Bottle

- Exercise Mat

- 5 to 15 lb. Weights

- Stability Ball

- Lots of Energy

- Gym Boss Timer (Optional)

I love my Gymboss Timer and use it all the time. They come in all sorts of fun colors.

Week Three
Exercises

ABS	REPS	SETS
AB In & Outs	15-20	2-3
Side Lying Leg Raise & Oblique Squeeze	15-20	2-3
Kill The Ants	15-20	2-3

CIRCUIT #1	REPS	SETS	WEIGHT
Stationary Lunges w. Shoulder Side Raise	10 / Leg	2-3	5-15 lbs.
1 Legged Back Row & Back Fly	10 / Leg	2-3	5-15 lbs.
Angled Out Bicep Curls & Calf Raises	20	2-3	5-15 lbs.
1/2 Burpees	30 sec.	2-3	Body Weight

CIRCUIT #2	REPS	SETS	WEIGHT
Pendulum Lunges	10 / Leg	2-3	5-15 lbs.
Curtsey Lunge w. Upright Shoulder Row	15	2-3	5-15 lbs.
Stability Ball Hamstring Curls & Pulses	15 15 Pulses	2-3	Body Weight
Downward Dog Heel Kicks	30 sec.	2-3	Body Weight

CIRCUIT #3	REPS	SETS	WEIGHT
Push Ups on the Ball	15	2-3	Body Weight
Squat with Rear Kick & Front Shoulder Raise	15	2-3	5-15 lbs.
1 Legged Sissy Squats	15 / leg	2-3	5-15 lbs.
Jump Rope	30 sec.	2-3	Body Weight

Cardio Program

20-Minute HIIT Cardio (High Intensity Interval Training)

I love High Intensity Training, because you get a big bang for your cardio buck and you know I like to get it in and get it done! You can do this on any cardio equipment or even outside walking, sprinting or running. You will get your heart pumping quickly. Challenge yourself, make it a game and you will have more fun.

Cardio Instructions:

Doing the extra cardio in addition to your circuit workouts will help you to burn fat faster. Keep in mind the workouts I gave you are heart pumping workouts. So if you don't have the time to add in 20 minutes of cardio it's OK. Do cardio on your non-circuit days.

Example of HIIT Interval Training

Treadmill or Elliptical

5 minute warm up

Interval Portion

1 minute increase resistance & speed on machine

1 minute reduce resistance & speed = recovery time

1 minute increase resistance & speed on machine

1 minute reduce resistance and speed = recovery time

Repeat the interval sequence 3-4 times

3 minute cool down

Outdoors:

Try 2 minutes of walking, then walk briskly for 30 seconds and then jog/sprint for 30 seconds; keep alternating. Include a cool down.

For moderate-intensity physical activity, a person's target heart rate should be 50% to 70% of his or her maximum heart rate. This maximum rate is based on the person's age. An estimate of a person's maximum age-related heart rate can be obtained by subtracting the person's age from 220. For example, for a 40-year-old person, the estimated maximum age-related heart rate would be calculated as

220 - 40 years = 180 beats per minute (bpm). Then 50% and 70% levels would be:

50% level: 180 x 0.50 = 90 bpm, and 70% level: 180 x 0.70 = 126 bpm

Exercises Explained: Workout 3

ABS

ABS In & Outs

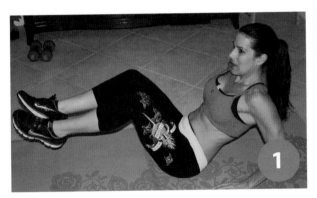 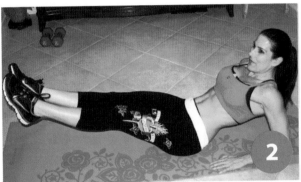

Lean back onto forearms. Lift legs up and crunch them to center, extend and repeat. Feel your abs working.

Side Lying Leg Raise & Oblique AB Squeeze

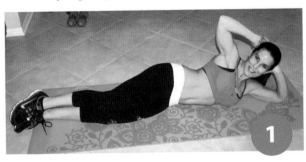 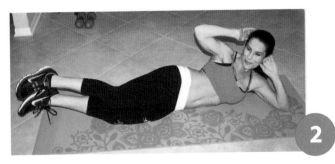

Lying on your side with hands behind your head. Gently lift feet off the floor and lift upper body to crunch toward your center and squeeze. Repeat on both sides of body.

ABS Kill The Ants Obliques

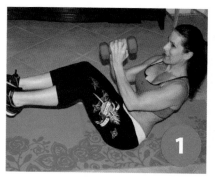 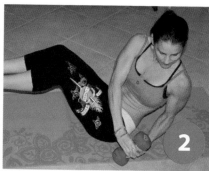 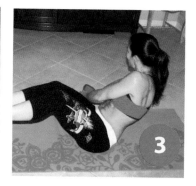

Lift feet off floor (beginners keep them on the ground) hold weight with both hands. Lean to the left; touch weight to floor, lean to the right, touch weight to the floor. Repeat.

CIRCUIT 1

Stationary Lunges With Shoulder Side Raise

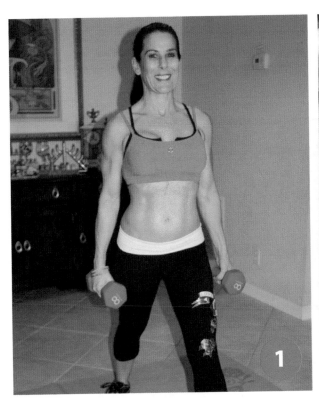 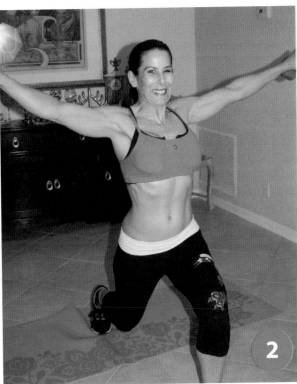

Lunge with your left foot forward and lower your body down. While in the lunge position raise your arms up to the sides. Lower weights back down to your sides. Keeping your feet stationary raise your body back up. Repeat this stationary lunge side raise combination for 10 reps. Switch to your right leg and repeat for 10 more reps.

1 Legged Back Row & Back Fly

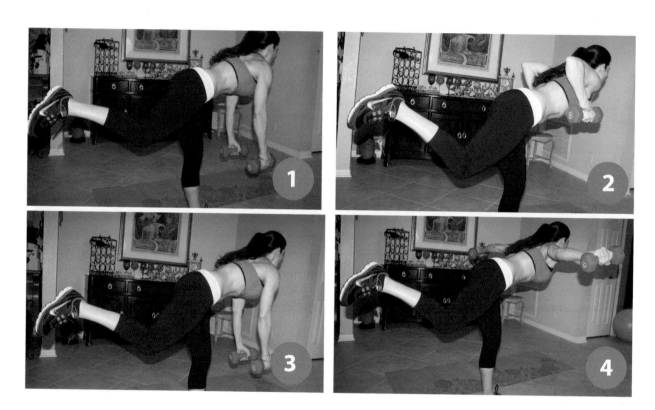

This is a great move for the back. Balance on one leg, pull your arms up to your sides and squeeze. Return to start and then bring arms out wide to the sides and squeeze. Burn baby burn.

Angled Out Bicep Curls & Calf Raises

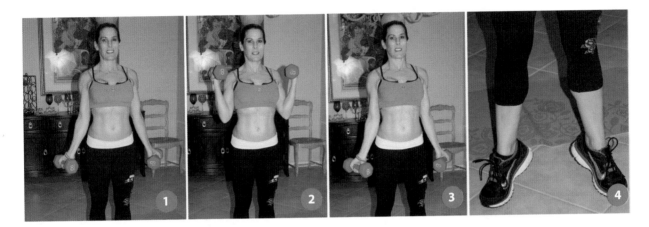

Stand with feet hip width apart. Palms facing upward to ceiling , arms angled out to the side of body. Perform a full bicep curl, Then, raise onto your tippy toes and lower. Repeat.

1/2 Burpees

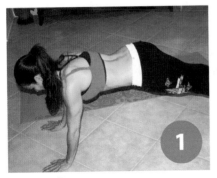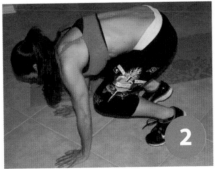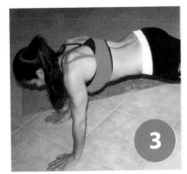

Start in the push up position, hop and bring feet toward knees, jump back repeat.

CIRCUIT 2

Pendulum Lunges

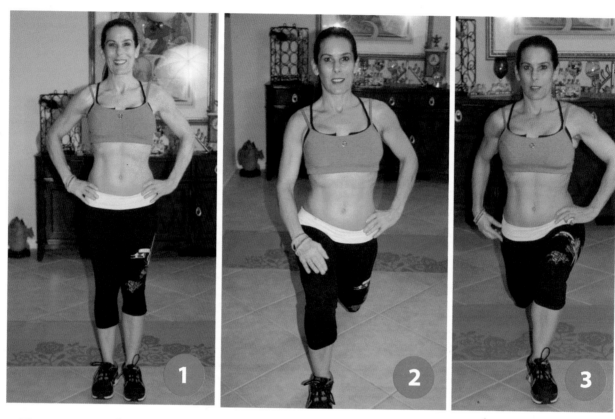

There are great for the thighs. Lunge forward and then sweep leg backward and lunge backward. Return to starting position.

Curtsey Lunge with Upright Shoulder Row

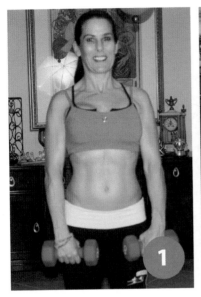 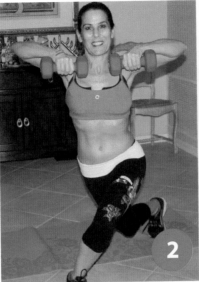 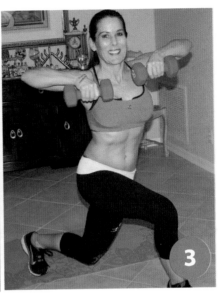

You can use a step in your house or a weight bench. The height of the step will increase the intensity of the exercise. Step up with one leg, perform a bicep hammer curl, tap toe on step and return to floor.

Stability Ball Hamstring Curls & Pulses

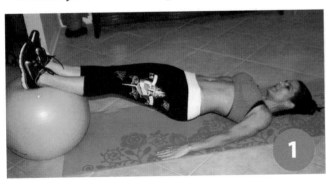 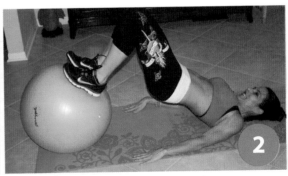

Place hands at side for balance, place feet on top of ball. Roll ball in toward your booty, then roll back out. When finished with reps add squeeze and pulses at end of set.

Downward Dog Heel Kicks

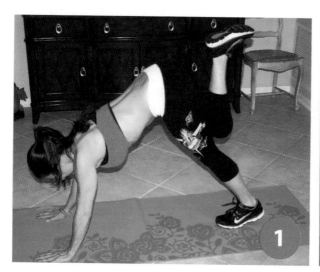 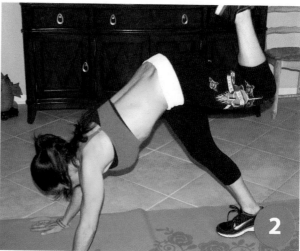

Place hands on floor, booty in the air. Start with one leg on the floor and one leg bent up to the ceiling. Alternate kicking up your legs in back of you.

CIRCUIT 3

Push Ups on the Ball

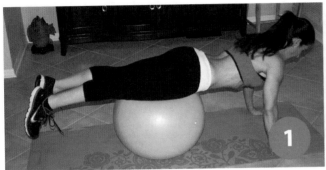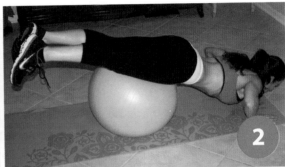

Push ups on the ball are a great way to build upper body strength. The farther you roll out the harder the exercise.

Squat with Rear Kick & Front Shoulder Raise

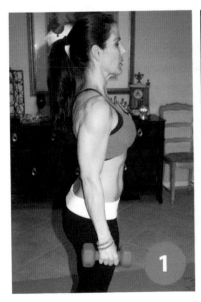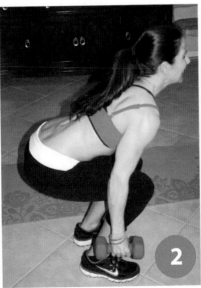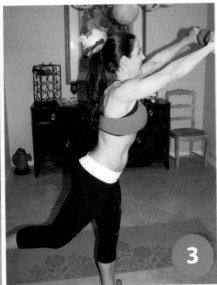

Squat down, and on the way back up balance on one leg, kicking the opposite leg behind you and squeezing the glutes. At the same time do a front shoulder raise. Return to center and do on opposite leg.

1 Legged Sissy Squats

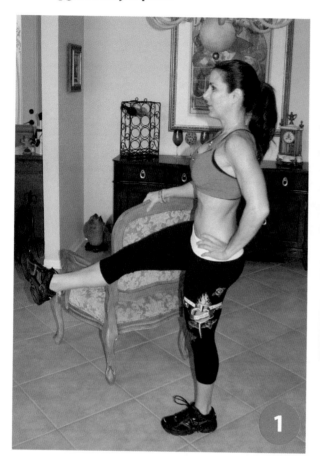

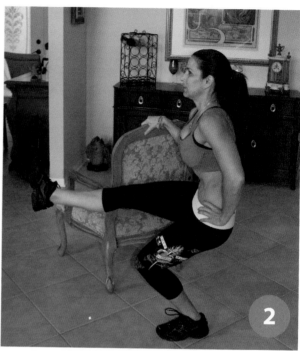

Jumping Rope

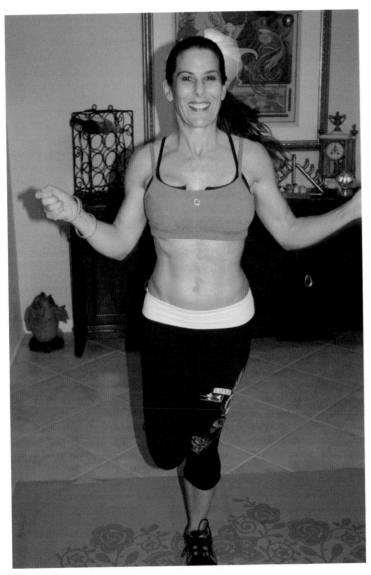

The beauty of this is you don't even need a jump rope. You can pretend and do all sorts of fancy tricks as long as you keep moving.

London GEM's Week Three

We are halfway there! I am so proud of how hard you are working and really taking the time to understand how your body works. This week we are going to learn how stress can be major contributor to extra body weight. Why getting a good nights rest is just as important as moving your body and how alkalizing the body can prevent health issues. Make sure to read about one of my favorite beauty secrets too!

Meet Cortisol The Fat Storage Hormone

I would like to introduce you to your "Stress Hormone". Her name is Cortisol.

She has a pretty name and has a very important job.

Cortisol works hard during times of fear or STRESS. Cortisol has some very cute nicknames "the death hormone," "the fat storage hormone." So cute, right?

Now let's talk about sweet Cortisol and STRESS… Cortisol is just doing her job day after day and she does it really well. Cortisol is made in your adrenal glands. In todays world we have a lot of stress and cortisol's job is to secrete more cortisol in times of stress.

EXAMPLES OF STRESS

- Work
- Relationships
- Family Issue
- Money Issues
- Overtraining the body
- Lack of sleep
- Poor Nutrition
- Worry, Fear, Anxiety
- TV News

Guess what? If our bodies are always in a constant state of STRESS then, sweet Cortisol is going to keep pumping out more Cortisol into your body.

Cortisol has some very cute nicknames: "the death hormone" and "the fat storage hormone".
Cute, right?

What does this mean? Well you know I am going to tell you, right?

EFFECTS OF ELEVATED CORTISOL

- Weight gain, especially in the abs and waistline
- Reduced growth hormone, testosterone, DHEA and estrogen
- Decreased bone density
- Decrease in muscle tissue

> *"The body always wants to remain in balance. It is your job to keep the balance by eating healthy, reducing stress, exercising and getting enough sleep"*

- Lowered immunity

- Lowers short-term memory and cognitive function

- Suppressed thyroid function

- Blood sugar imbalances

- Suppress DHEA, the "youth" hormone

Now lets talk blood sugar. We always strive to keep our blood sugar in balance by eating clean and natural foods and eating regularly throughout the day. But when the body is STRESSED constantly, Cortisol causes blood sugar to elevate, which can lead to an acidic condition. When our blood is in a higher acidic state this can lead to diseases such as cancer, heart disease and diabetes.

The body is all about balance and always wants to remain in balance. It is your job to keep the balance by eating healthy, reducing stress, exercising and getting enough sleep.

WAYS TO FIND YOUR BALANCE

Eat Clean – Eating clean means eating foods as close to Mother Nature as possible. Organic is always the best choice. Eat a balanced diet of healthy fats, proteins, fresh fruits and veggies. Packaged food and sugar are the enemy.

Exercising - Exercising is a great stress reliever for the body. It also can improve your mood, boost energy, help fight disease, promote better sleep and can just be fun.

Exercise can also be a stress on the body. Your workouts should invigorate you but not stress the body too much. Over training or over obsessing about working out also cause an imbalance in the body adding to the stress and cortisol level. Remember BALANCE is the key.

Sleep – This is a big one for most of us. We are up late watching TV or on the computer, which stimulates the brain. Caffeine that is consumed during the day is still in our blood stream many hours later. So just be aware that afternoon cup of coffee, soda or energy drink will still be with you when your head hits the pillow hours later.

STRESS REDUCING SUGGESTIONS

- Turn off the TV at night and read instead
- Try the essential oil Lavender; it is calming and relaxing
- When was the last time you soaked in the bathtub?
- Drink less caffeine
- Try meditation
- Listen to relaxing music
- Dim the lights before you go to bed to set the tone
- Talk with a friend
- Laugh often and laugh hard
- Be grateful
- Smile
- Eat a balanced diet

In conclusion, Cortisol is only doing her job and you need to do your job and live in balance as much as possible.

Are You Living in a Toxic Body?

For those of you who don't know, I love fitness! I enjoy exercising and the feeling I get from feeling strong and in control of my body. But what you might not know about me is that fitness is my hobby.

Nutrition and how the body works are my passion.

I graduated from the largest nutrition school in the country, Integrative Nutrition. But even before that, actually since I can remember, I have been studying nutrition and it's effects on the body. I have even been my own science experiment, living vegetarian, raw, vegan and even the bodybuilding lifestyle.

I have been to raw food retreats and learned to create the most amazing dishes, done fasts and cleanses, juiced wheatgrass and studied reflexology and aromatherapy. I even have penned my own juicing Ebook, The 7-Day Goddess Juice Feast.

I have earned the name the Organic Green Goddess, and am here to share with you how to take care of your body the healthy green natural way, so lets do it! To Alkalize or not to Alkalize? Now that's a silly question

A little lesson here on your bodies PH. The PH scale goes from 0 to 14. O is pure acid and 14 is pure alkaline, 7 is neutral.

The human body's blood stream is between 7.35 to 7.45 PH. This is a very small range. Our blood is just slightly alkaline. The body needs it to stay in this very tight range.

What happens when the blood becomes too acidic? Disease starts to set in. If the blood acidity falls as little as to 7 PH it can be life threatening.

The Acidic Lifestyle

In today's world with all the processed foods, drive through restaurants and social get-togethers, over acidification of our bodies is a HUGE problem. Combine that with lack of exercise and it is no wonder we are having all sorts of health issues.

An acidic body is a breeding ground for bacteria, fungi, yeast and even cancer cells. Some things that cause an acidic body are processed foods, medications, lack of exercise and stress.

Healthy cells love oxygen; cancer cells can't live in an environment that is "oxygen happy". Cancer cells live in dark dingy places that lack oxygen, an ACIDIC BODY…. And they also LOVE sugar!!!

Ok, so how do we make our bodies more ALKALIZED?

Well, I thought you would never ask. It is easy to start doing right now:

- Stay away from processed foods, artificial flavors, colors & preservatives
- Juice with green juices (full of oxygen & living enzymes)
- Exercise oxygenates the cells in the body
- Get a good night sleep.
- Avoid processed SUGAR at all cost
- Eat Organic whenever possible
- Reduce the amount of toxic chemicals you put on your body
- Avoid drinking from plastic bottles
- Drink filtered or alkalized water

Soda is extremely acid forming. It ages the body and helps to create the perfect acidic environment for the body's cells to give way to cancer and other harmful diseases. SODA has a pH of 2.3; once it is ingested, your body has to give the acidic soda all of its energy to try and balance the harmful effect taking place within the body.

Now, I want you to go run and pull out your juicer or blender and make a beautiful green juice or smoothie and oxygenate your body. Think of your cells dancing around in happiness as you give them a tall glass of "GREEN LOVE" and start to alkalize the body.

Remember, every cell in your body is made of what you put in and on it.

Raw Coconut Oil Kitchen, Bathroom and Bedroom!

I love RAW coconut oil. I have a jar in my kitchen and a jar in my bathroom. That's right! The benefits of raw coconut oil are many. Coconut oil has gotten a very bad rap, but did you know the stories they are telling are about hydrogenated coconut oil? The kind they put in candy, and cookies to have a shelf life of about a million years.

Raw coconut oil (RCO) is a gift from Mother Nature to be treasured. RCO is a medium chain triglyceride that the body uses immediately as an energy source. It does not get stored as fat.

Some of the many health benefits of RCO:

- Assists in weight loss
- Helps the body to eliminate parasites, fungus and viruses
- Has been shown to be beneficial for the thyroid
- Helps to balance hormones
- Helps to improve digestion
- Keeps the skin soft and helps prevent premature aging

I spread it on my sprouted grain toast and use it to cook with. Because coconut oil is mainly a saturated fat, it is stable and the heat of cooking does not create a free radical frenzy.

Coconut oil is liquid at room temperature and will turn to a solid when cold. You can use it in place of any oil and do not need to change a recipe when using it. So go bake some healthy muffins and enjoy.

I use coconut oil on my body as a moisturizer. There are no added chemicals like the toxic lotions you buy in the stores and I love the smell and my skin is so soft. Careful if you have pets because they love it and will try to lick it off you.

No worries because it is good for them too. Try it as a deep conditioning treatment on the ends of your hair; a little goes a long way.

Remember, I said coconut oil in the bedroom. That's right ladies, sometimes things may not run as smoothly as we may want. Coconut oil is a natural, healthy and safe lubricant for the bedroom.

Try a massage with your husband or boyfriend using coconut oil. Your body will eat it up, your skin will be smoother than ever and not to mention the quality time you will be spending together. Go give it a try!

Thank you coconut oil!

Exercise 101
Week 4

How on earth did we get to week four already? I am excited and sad that we are already here at the same time. The fact you are here means that you were true to yourself and kept your word and did not give up. How are you feeling? I am really proud of you and you should be very proud of yourself. You followed through, you did something just for you!

Your clothes are looser now, your digestion and metabolism are running at full speed and you have lost your addiction to sugar and carbohydrates. You have learned a lot about your Hot and Healthy Body and how to keep it fit and healthy for life. You learned that loving yourself and speaking to yourself with kind motivating words and thoughts are the only way to talk to yourself from this day forward.

You now know how great circuit workouts are and how to change them up to challenge your body and most important how to fit them into your schedule. Done are the days of endless cardio and getting nowhere. It's not how much time you spend exercising that is important but doing something each week and making the commitment to yourself to move your body. Try changing up your fitness routine and adding in new things so you don't get bored. Try a Zumba or Pilates class, maybe a bike ride or a nice walk with your main man.

Your new journaling and goal setting skills will be something that you practice for a lifetime. Putting your thoughts and feelings down on paper helps you to see where you may need to make some tweaks or adjustments to keep you on your Hot and Healthy path. You will be reaching your goals and always continuing to strive to meet new ones. Life is much more rewarding when you have goals to work towards.

Taking the time to take care of yourself from now on is top priority in your life. Done are the days of putting everyone else first and hoping there will be time left for you. When we take the time to take care and nourish not only our bodies but our inner goddess we have so much more to offer our family and friends. We are happier and we are healthier.

The Hot and Healthy Body is a long term commitment not only to yourself but to your family and friends. It does not end here; it does not end, ever. We are always learning and growing as individuals. Now that you have all this wonderful information, it is your duty to help spread the gift of health and wellness. If you are able to touch just one life think of all the lives that could be changed if we each helped just one person. Personally, that is what this health and fitness journey is truly about for me. It may have started with my "WHY' of losing weight and getting into shape but what it turned into was really a movement of creating hundreds and thousands of Hot and Healthy Bodies across the globe. Together we are stronger.

This may be the last week in the Hot and Healthy Body program but it is just the beginning for you and your new healthy body. Keep going, keep using and referring back to all the principles and guidelines I have shared with you. We both know they work when you follow them. They make sense because they are based on how your body truly works. Remember if you get a little off your path, just jump right back on.

You have a brand new Hot and Healthy workout this week! Get ready to really challenge yourself and see how far you have come. Your strength has increased, your shape is changing. You are feeling tighter and toned. It is just going to get better and better now that you have all the tools you need.

This week we are going to discuss how to further reduce inflammations by taking out or rotating foods that may be causing your body to show signs of inflammation. We will discuss the importance of what we put not only in our bodies but on our skin and how it affects our weight loss. We will talk about cellulite, why we get it and ways to reduce it's appearance.

Week 4 Check List:

- Read your Goals everyday

- Journal your food every day

- Journal your thoughts and feelings each day

- Drink up to 64 oz. of quality water

- Perform your circuit workout 3 to 4 times a week

- Mark your workouts with an X on your success calendar

- Weigh yourself and take measurements once a week

- Remove "Franken Foods" from your home

- Add in extra cardio to speed up results

- Nurture Your Inner Goddess by doing something special just for you

- Add a green drink or smoothie to your nutrition plan

- Find one new healthy recipe a week to try

- Enjoy the goddess body you have today and live with passion

The Workouts:

The workouts start with 3 AB exercises. I love starting with the ABS because it is a great warm up for the whole body. Next you will move into your circuits. There are three circuits in each workout. Run through the AB circuit before moving on the whole body circuits.

Depending on your ability level run through each circuit one to three times before moving on to the next circuit. Rest when you need it and build up your strength.

Every exercise can be performed at the beginner, intermediate and advanced level. Increase your range of motion, tempo and weight used to increase the difficulty. Challenge yourself and make the mind muscle connection. Don't just do the movements, feel the movements.

Doing the whole routine once should take you about 20 minutes, running through the circuits twice should take you about 40 minutes, running through all the circuits 3 times should take you 60 minutes.

What You Need

This is a list of the equipment you are going to need for your Hot and Healthy Workouts. The beauty of the workouts is that you can do them at home or in the gym. Print them out and take them with you or save them to your iPhone or iPad. I have done all these workouts myself and use them with my personal training clients, so I know they work.

· Water Bottle

· Exercise Mat

· 5 to 15 lb. Weights

· Stability Ball

· Lots of Energy

· Gym Boss Timer (Optional)

I love my Gymboss Timer and use it all the time. They come in all sorts of fun colors.

Week Four Exercises

ABS	REPS	SETS
20 Toe Tap Abs	20	2-3
Fold It Like A Lawn Chair ABS	10 / side	2-3
In & Out ABS	20	2-3

CIRCUIT #1	REPS	SETS	WEIGHT
Stability Ball Chest Press & Chest Flyes	15 Presses 15 Flyes	2-3	5-15 lbs.
Push Ups On The Ball	failure	2-3	Body Weight
Squat w. Front Kicks	15	2-3	5-15 lbs.
Power Jumping Jacks	15	2-3	Body Weight

CIRCUIT #2	REPS	SETS	WEIGHT
20 Regular Squats	20	2	0-10 lbs.
20 Half Squats	20	2	0-10 lbs.
20 Side Kick Squats	20	2	0-10 lbs.

CIRCUIT #2 (ctd.)	REPS	SETS	WEIGHT
20 Front Kick Squats	20	2	0-10lbs
20 Rear Kick Squats	20	2	0-10lbs

CIRCUIT #3	REPS	SETS	WEIGHT
Triceps Kick Back & Overhead Shoulder Press	15	2-3	5-15 lbs.
Walking "Laura London" Lunges	10 Walking 10 Stationary 10 Walking 10 Stationary	2-3	5-15 lbs.
Standing Back Row & Back Fly	15	2-3	5-15 lbs.
High Knee Slaps	30 sec.	2-3	Body Weight

Cardio Program

20-Minute HIIT Cardio (High Intensity Interval Training)

I love High Intensity Training. You get a big bang for your cardio buck and you know I like to get it in and get it done! You can do this on any cardio equipment or even outside walking, sprinting or running. You will get your heart pumping quickly. Challenge yourself, make it a game and you will have more fun.

Cardio Instructions:

Doing the extra cardio in addition to your circuit workouts will help you to burn fat faster. Keep in mind the workouts I gave you are heart pumping workouts. So if you don't have the time to add in 20 minutes of cardio it's ok. Do cardio on your non circuit days.

Example of HIIT Interval Training

Treadmill or Elliptical

5 minute warm up

Interval Portion

1 minute increase resistance & speed on machine

1 minute reduce resistance & speed = recovery time

1 minute increase resistance & speed on machine

1 minute reduce resistance and speed = recovery time

Repeat the interval sequence 3-4 times

3 minute cool down

Outdoors:

Try 2 minutes of walking, then walk briskly for 30 seconds and then jog/sprint for 30 seconds. Keep alternating. Include a cool down.

For moderate-intensity physical activity, a person's target heart rate should be 50% to 70% of his or her maximum heart rate. This maximum rate is based on the person's age. An estimate of a person's maximum age-related heart rate can be obtained by subtracting the person's age from 220. For example, for a 40-year-old person, the estimated maximum age-related heart rate would be calculated as

220 - 40 years = 180 beats per minute (bpm). Then 50% and 70% levels would be:

50% level: 180 x 0.50 = 90 bpm, and 70% level: 180 x 0.70 = 126 bpm

Exercises Explained: Workout 4

ABS

Toe Tap Abs

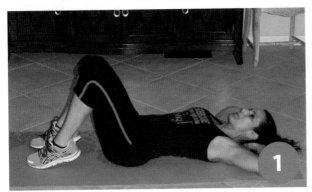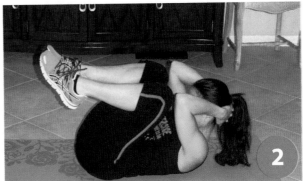

Feet close to booty, hands behind head. Crunch up, touching elbows to knees. Gently tap floor with toes, make sure to keep toes as close to the booty as possible. This makes the ABS work harder.

Fold It Like A Lawn Chair ABS

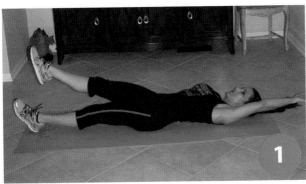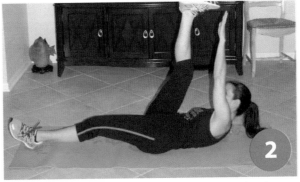

Reach opposite hand to opposite foot, reach up and meet in the middle. Feel the squeeze in the ABS. Extend back out but do not let hands or feet touch the floor. Complete reps on one side then move to the other side.

In & Out ABS

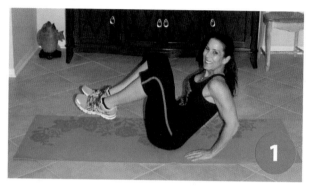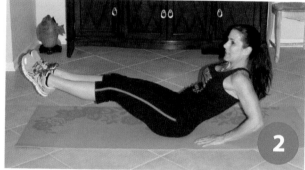

Lean back on hands pull legs towards body, then extend forward and lean back a little. Repeat.

CIRCUIT 1

Stability Ball Chest Press & Chest Flyes

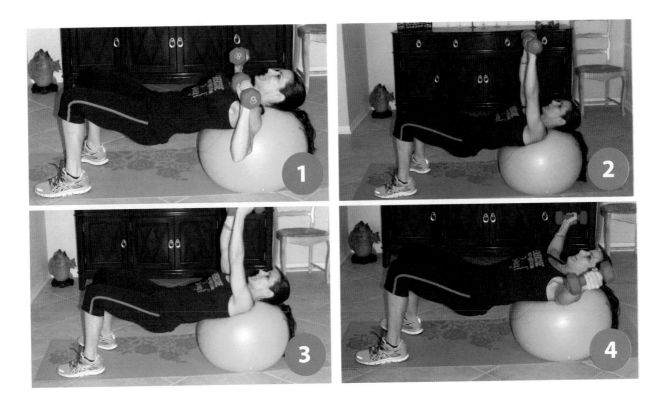

Push Ups on the Stability Ball

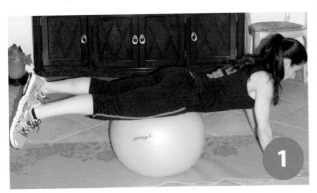
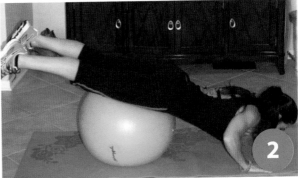

Squat with Front Kicks

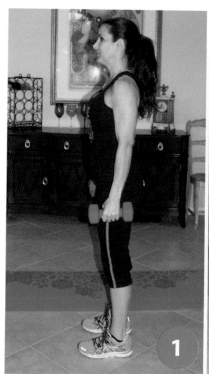
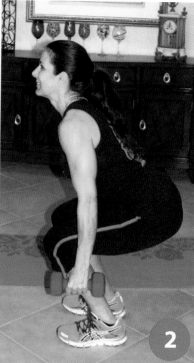
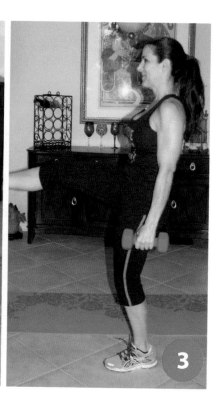

Power Jumping Jacks

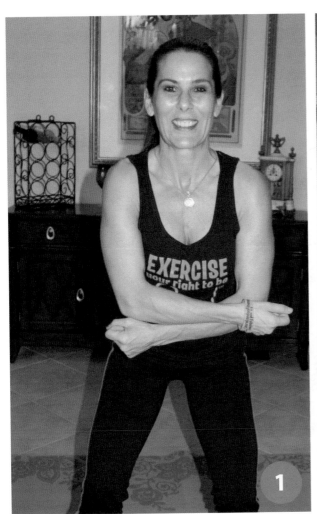
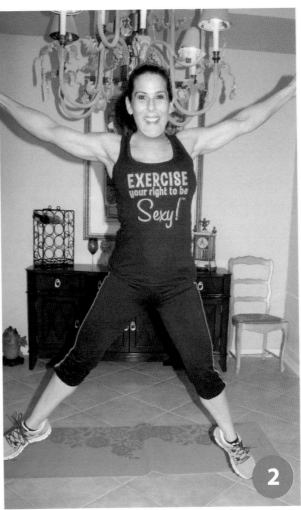

CIRCUIT 2

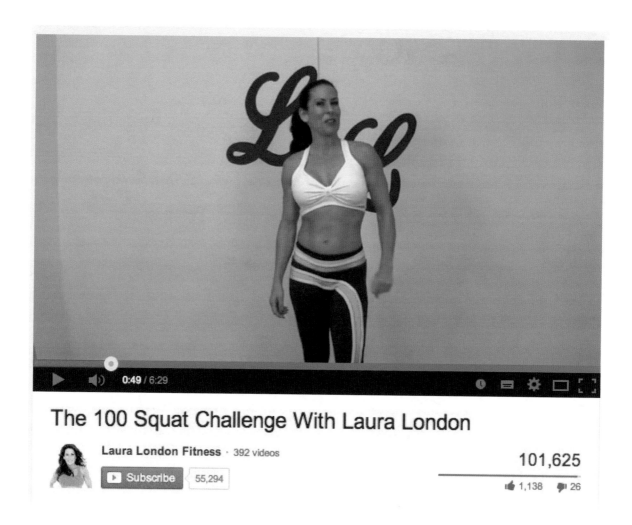

Watch the Video "The 100 Squat Challenge" at
https://www.youtube.com/watch?v=Xq-NCeUg1nU

CIRCUIT 3

Triceps Kick Back & Overhead Shoulder Press

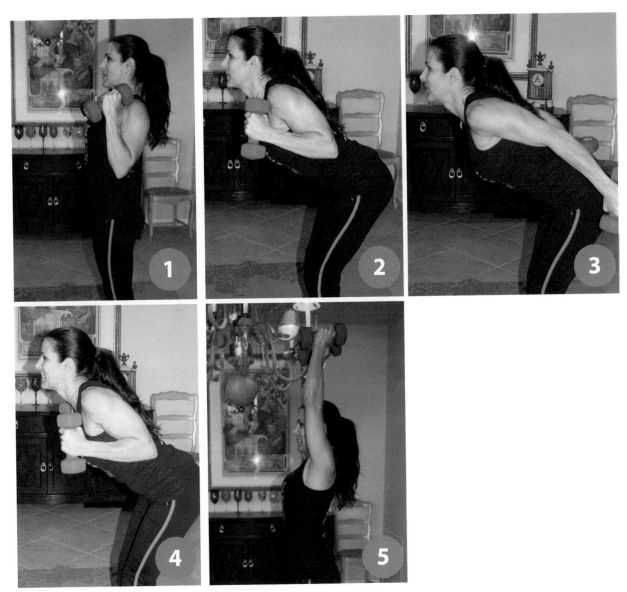

Bend forward, slight bend in the knee, pull weights to side of chest, extend elbows backward and return weights to starting position. Think of your elbows as a hinge. Stand up straight, do on overhead shoulder press, lower and then repeat.

Walking "Laura London" Lunges

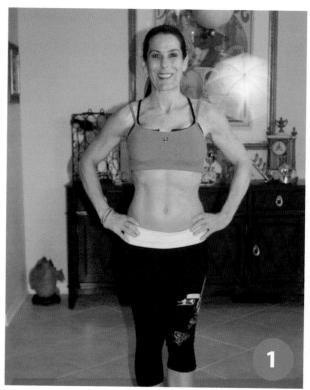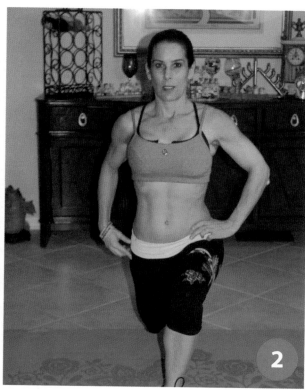

10 walking lunges, then do 10 stationary lunges (up & down) then 10 walking and 10 stationary lunges. Feel the London Burn in your quads. If 10 is too many start with 5 of each.

Standing Back Row & Back Fly

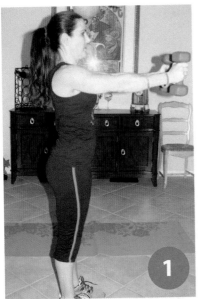
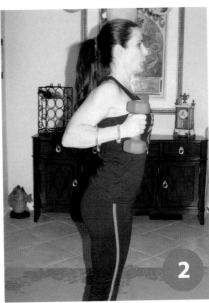
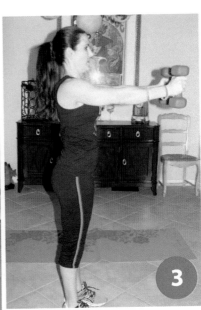

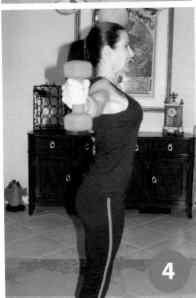

This is a multi movement exercise. Hold weights in front of you, palms facing each other. Row arms back and squeeze, return to starting position, fly arms out to sides, feel squeeze in back return to center. Repeat.

High Knee Slaps

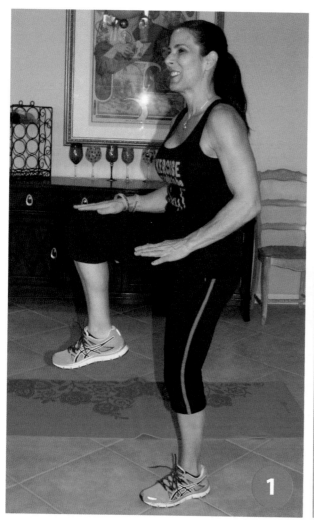 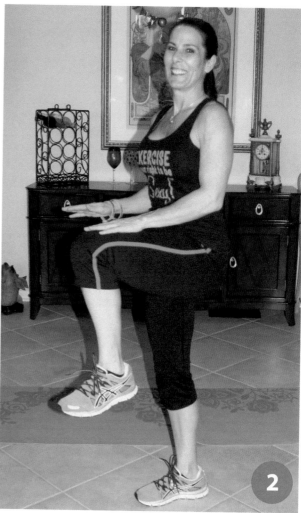

Great cardio, bring those knees up high and slap them, alternating legs with a hop.

London GEM's Week Four

This is the final week. You are well on your way to a Hot and Healthy Body now and I am so excited and happy for you. Learning to love the skin you are in today and forever. Week four is about understanding your own individual body and what truly works for you. Every body and everybody are different. Some people may thrive on a vegan or vegetarian nutrition plan and some might not. What I want you to understand is that there is no right or wrong just listening to what works best for your body type. We are also going to talk about the "C" word, cellulite. Plus, why the elimination diet can help you find food sensitivities that may be causing inflammation and halting your weight loss goals

Food Sensitivities - Listening to Your Body

You are the only you on this planet. Each body works and responds differently to different foods. When you write in your food journal note any signs or symptoms you may have after eating a certain food. Often an inability to lose weight is connected to inflammation caused by consuming foods that your body is intolerant of. The 30 days of healthy eating is your chance to understand what is creating inflammation in your body so that you can more easily and effectively decrease that inflammation, lose the weight, and ditch the diet forever.

Elimination Diet

The Elimination Diet involves removing specific foods for 7 days and then adding them back into your diet one at a time. Journal how you are feeling when you take out one of these foods and then when you add it back in for 2-3 days. You may find that you have a hidden food allergy that has been causing you issues that you never knew about.

> *"We all have different sensitivities, tune into them and notice how your body reacts when you eat certain foods."*

The 7 most common allergenic foods include:

- Soy
- Dairy
- Eggs
- Fish/shellfish
- Caffeine
- Wheat
- Nuts

"We are exposed to toxins in the air we breathe and the environment around us daily. Helping the body to detox is important and very helpful in weight loss."

We all have different sensitivities, tune into them and notice how your body reacts when you eat certain foods.

"You need to listen to your body, because it's listening to you"

-Phillip C. McGraw

Goddess Beauty You Are What You Put On Your Skin

I touched on the raw coconut oil I use to moisturize my skin. But that is just the beginning of what I am going to share with you. First let me ask you a question.

If a doctor can put a birth control patch on the outside of a woman's arm to keep her from getting pregnant, where do you think all the chemicals (that you can't even pronounce) in the fragrant and colorful lotions you use are going? Humm, got you thinking didn't I?

I will tell you where they are going. Into your skin, into your vital organs, and into your fat cell and do you know what they are doing inside your body?

You know I am going to tell you, don't you? They are throwing your body off balance, messing with your hormones and are just plain toxic. I know they smell so good, but from now on I want you to understand what you are putting on and in your body. Years and years of using these products adds up to a very heavy toxic load.

The body is very sensitive and also very smart, when it is having a very hard time staying in balance it lets you know. The skin is our largest organ that gets rid of toxins. How?

Well think about it, the body can't talk like you and I can. So it sends us signals, signals in the form of pimples, rashes, eczema, joint aches, puffy eyes and all sorts of other signals.

It is screaming, HELP! I am out of balance. Eat better quality food, drink water, stop using all the chemical laden beauty and cleaning products. I CAN'T TAKE IT ANY MORE".

Where Did All This Cellulite Come From?

Many women even famous celebrities struggle with cellulite. We don't want it, but how do we make it go away or diminish the look of those not so attractive bumps and lumps?

There are three main causes of cellulite. Guess which is at the top of the list?

1. The toxins from junk foods and chemicals that you put in and on your body. There are serious hormone disrupters. Remember toxins that come into the body are surrounded like space invaders, grabbed and pushed as far away from our precious organs. The body wants to protect those vital organs at all costs.

We are exposed to toxins in the air we breathe and the environment around us daily. So helping the body to detox on a regular basis is important and very helpful in weight loss.

2. The second reason for cellulite is too much body fat. This is really related to number one. The more fat we have, generally the more Franken Foods we are eating, the more cellulite one may have. Our fat cells get fatter when they are storing toxins in them.

3. Lack of muscle tissue and loose skin. Having muscle make the skin nice and tight and pushes the fat cells up so cellulite is not seen as much. Have you ever seen a model that is thin but yet, still she has bumpy thighs and booty? This is because she is lacking muscle tone underneath. So I want you to do 50 booty squeezes right now! Just kidding. But adding muscle toning exercises is really important in decreasing the look of cellulite.

There are other factors that go into why one person has more or less cellulite such as heredity and birth origin. But don't worry, I am working on a cellulite book as we speak where I will go more in depth.

So now that I have your attention. All I am trying to get across to you is to start making better choices in your beauty products, read the labels, see what ingredients are in the products and ask yourself do I want to use this on my body or can I find a better quality product? Is this for my higher good?

KEY TOXIC WORDS TO LOOK FOR

In Your Health & Beauty Products

Parabens

Butyl Acetate

Diethanolamine (DEA)

Sodium Lauryl Sulfate

Fragrance

Propylene Glycol

Butylated Hydroxyanisole (BHA)

FDC Artificial Colors

Triclosan

Nitrates

There are so many chemicals that are being put into our health and beauty product and our little innocent babies products.

I could write a whole book on this issue, because this is how strongly I feel about this issue. What a great idea!

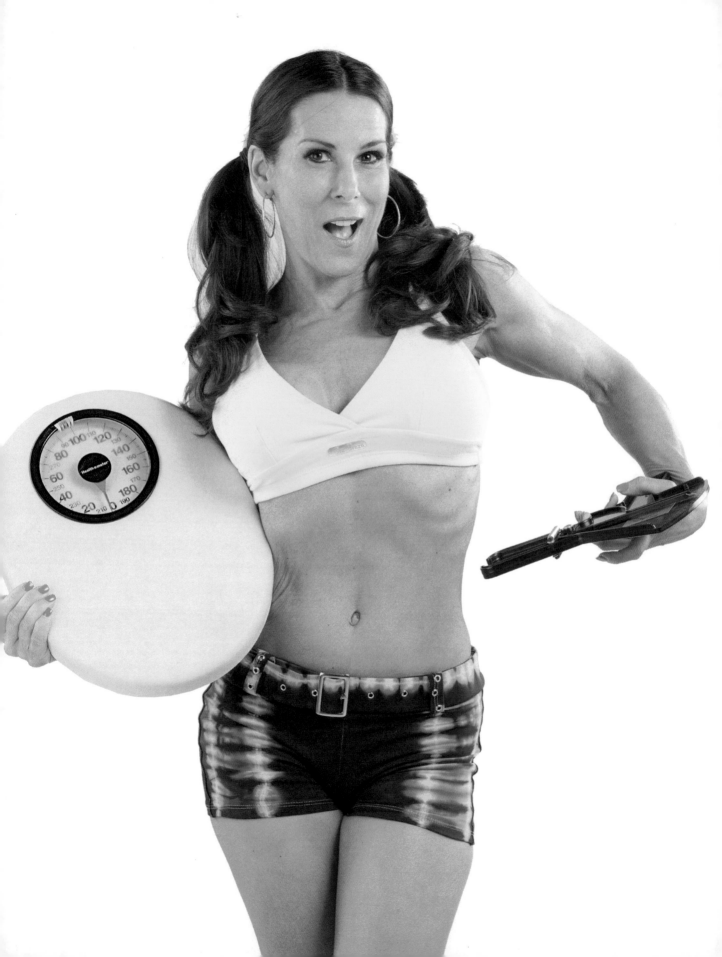

Resources

Hot and Healthy Body Journal

www.HotAndHealthyBody.com/journal

Visit the link above to download your complimentary Hot and Healthy Nutrition and Fitness Journal!

Laura London Fitness Newsletter

www.LauraLondonFitness.com

Get on the list! I send free recipes, health and fitness tips, and you also get a copy of my guide "10 Surprising Secrets to Getting Fit and Fabulous in Your 40's with a family".

7 Days To Goddess Slim

www.GoddessSlim.com

Are you tired of living in a body that does not feel like yours? Are you ready to let your inner beautiful Goddess shine and take on the world? The 7 Days to Goddess Slim is a Jump Start Program that I designed to break your carbohydrate and sugar cravings and get your metabolism functioning like a red race car in the Indy 500.

7-Day Goddess Juice Feast

www.7DayGoddessJuiceFeast.com

This is the easiest Juice Feast because there are no crazy rules. It's based on you, your body and drinking high quality nourishing juices. Over 30 juice feast recipes and photos. It's a great place to start if you have ever thought of juicing for one day or 7 days. Recharge, energize and give your goddess body the love it deserves. 7 Days to vibrant health, clear skin and abundant energy.

Institute for Integrative Nutrition

www.integrativenutrition.com

Create a career out of your passion for health, wellness, and helping others. Invigorate your health, live your passion and design a life you love. It's one of the best decisions I ever made. Let them know Laura sent you!

Real Talk Real Women the Book

www.RealTalkRealWomen.net

100 of the top health and fitness professionals sharing 100 life -changing chapters - all in one book.   A book that teaches about self-love, persistence, success, balance and making a difference. Find out what supermodels,fitness guru's, elite athletes, Ph Ds & female CEO's have in common.

If there is just one book you read before the end of this year, make it this one! I know you are going to love it Plus I am in the book, chapter #97 "Making a Difference In the World".

Purium Health Products

www.mypurium.com/lauralondon

Purium's mission is to help you look, feel and perform like a much younger person with organic and non-GMO super foods. Together we can educate and support our families in "The Real Food Revolution". Be part of the million Mom movement and let's take back our food. With Purium you will enjoy the most potent, whole food, raw food, live food, green food, super-concentrated, highly alkalized, organic, vegan, super-food products.

BlendTec Blender

www.lauralondonfitness.com/blog/blendtec

Don't be without the best blender in the world if you are serious about clean whole food living. I use my Blendtec blender everyday and would not be without it.

GymBoss Timer

http://bit.ly/GymBossLauraLondon

The GYMBOSS is a small, easy to use, repeating interval timer. This multi-use timer has many versatile functions that make it beneficial to virtually any type of exercise program.

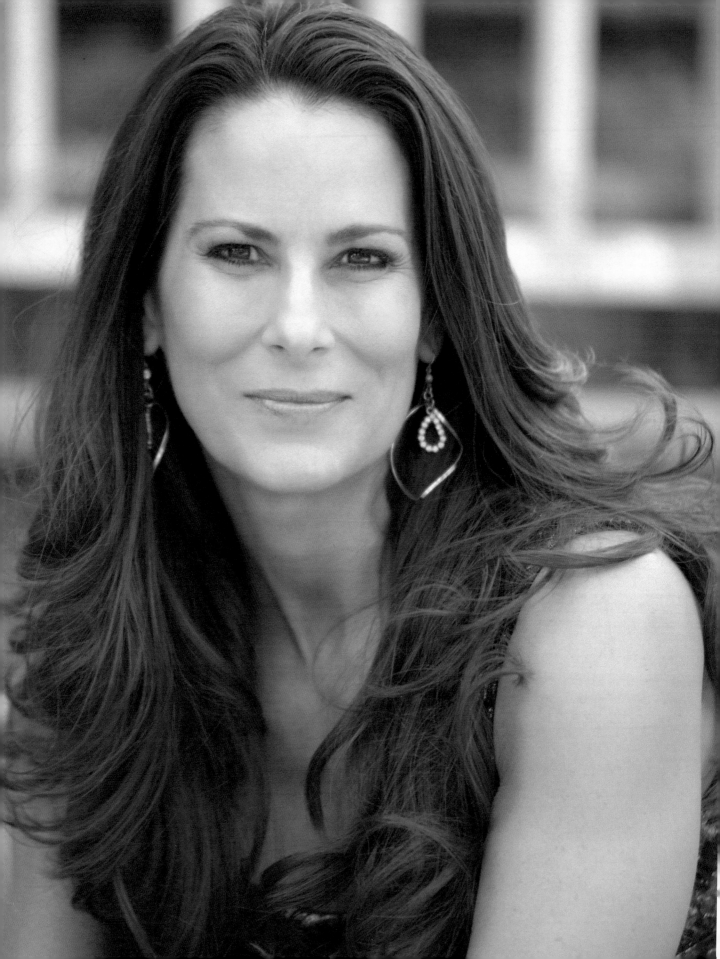

About the Author

Laura London is a Board Certified Holistic Health Counselor, Nationally Certified Personal Trainer as well as an author and a 40's fitness & lifestyle model. Laura's focus is on what you gain by becoming a healthier version of yourself. Gaining confidence, pleasure, feeling great in your own skin and having a fit and healthy body. While at the same time re-discovering your inner Goddess and letting her shine from the inside out.

Laura found herself, like many other woman in their 40's tired, out of shape, overweight and wondering what had happened to her once healthy lifestyle. She took action, changed not only her diet but also, the course of her life through natural holistic living. Laura is here to help you build a body you love and a life you love, today!

Laura has dedicated her life to healthy eating and fitness. Laura's passion is to educate others to look and feel their best at any age and she shares her own remedies to bring health and vibrancy back into your life.

Laura is a published fitness model and has been featured in Planet Muscle Magazine, Natural Muscle Magazine as well as being featured in fitness DVD's. Laura is published in the popular fitness book Real Talk Real Woman. Laura has also studied reflexology, raw food preparation and is an essential oils instructor. She is a wife of over twenty years and a mother of three.

To learn more about Laura's nutritional courses, events she's hosting and custom programs, visit www.LauraLondonFitness. com and follow her on Facebook, YouTube and Twitter.